parent
like a
pediatrician

ALL

THE FACTS,

NONE

OF THE FEAR

Rebekah Diamond, MD

CITADEL PRESS

Kensington Publishing Corp.

www.kensingtonbooks.com

parent
like a
pediatrician

CITADEL PRESS BOOKS are published by

Kensington Publishing Corp.
119 West 40th Street
New York, NY 10018

PUBLISHER'S NOTE

This book is sold to readers with the understanding that while the publisher aims to inform, enlighten, and provide accurate general information regarding the subject matter covered, the publisher is not engaged in providing medical, psychological, financial, legal, or other professional services. If the reader needs or wants professional advice or assistance, the services of an appropriate professional should be sought. Case studies featured in this book are composites based on the author's years of practice and do not reflect the experiences of any individual person.

All Kensington titles, imprints, and distributed lines are available at special quantity discounts for bulk purchases for sales promotions, premiums, fund-raising, educational, or institutional use. Special book excerpts or customized printings can also be created to fit specific needs. For details, write or phone the office of the Kensington sales manager: Kensington Publishing Corp., 119 West 40th Street, New York, NY 10018, attn: Sales Department; phone 1-800-221-2647.

CITADEL PRESS and the Citadel logo are Reg. U.S. Pat. & TM Off.

ISBN: 978-0-8065-4163-1

First trade paperback printing: October 2022

10 9 8 7 6 5 4 3 2 1

Printed in the United States of America

First electronic edition: October 2022

ISBN: 978-0-8065-4164-8

To P and B, with all my love

CONTENTS

Contents

INTRODUCTION

The internet broke parenting.

In the "good old days," parents followed a few basic pediatrician-approved rules—send your kid to school, give them healthy food, say "I love you"—and felt confident that they were raising their children right. But today, even the basics have become needlessly complicated.

As a new parent, you'll have access to more information than ever before—but you will also have more reasons than ever to doubt it. Modern parenting advice comes from two very different and often-conflicting sources. On the one hand, you have the "mommy blogs," filled with anecdotes that are personal and accessible. On the other hand, there are the official pediatric organizations (such as the American Academy of Pediatrics, Centers for Disease Control and Prevention, and World Health Organization), which present a never-ending list of rules and regulations that, while based on good science, often ignore the realities of parenting and the everyday challenges that stand in the way of following rigid guidelines.

As a pediatrician-in-training—before I became a mother—I recited these rules to parents and expected them to do everything as outlined: minimize screen time (this was before the WHO had adopted its latest zero-tolerance policy); breastfeed exclusively; never, ever, co-sleep; and, most important,

1

to remember that the internet, filled with unscientific advice, should never be trusted.

But when I became a mom, my world was turned upside down. I immediately violated many of the very rules I had issued as a pediatrician. When my daughter had trouble latching, I gave her formula. When she got sick, or even a bit fussier than usual, I turned on the TV and let the screen tag in as the babysitter. And after years of preaching the importance of structured family meals, I even found myself hosting "toddler picnics," when on particularly rushed mornings I shared breakfast with my nine-month-old, served on paper towels, sitting on the floor, to maximize efficiency and minimize mess. I couldn't believe that for years I had been so black-and-white with my patients, rigidly defending guidelines and best practices I now know are impossible to follow perfectly.

At work, I swapped war stories with fellow pediatrician parents, confessing how I had forgotten to brush my infant's teeth for the past week, or had served a bottle of breast milk left on the counter an hour after its expiration. All my coworkers had made similar choices, also shocked that they'd ever been so rigid in their recommendations. From mild violations like extending pacifier use to the cardinal sin of modifying rigid "safe sleep" practices, every pediatrician mother admitted to making compromises and breaking strict AAP rules.

I also did the unthinkable: I started reading mommy blogs.

I was both validated and shocked. I understood immediately why so many parents turn to these funny and humanizing websites as their sole source of information. "Guilt-free" parenting essays, blogs, and social media accounts appear as lifeboats in an ocean of stressful, unrealistic expectations. When the American Academy of Pediatrics commands that babies sleep in their parents' room for a whole year on the same handout that promotes excellent and important safe sleep practices, it's easy to simply lose trust and turn elsewhere.

But "guilt-free" parenting isn't the answer. The science is lacking, and the suggestions can be downright dangerous. Some bloggers, seeking free products, plug unsafe items. At their worst, popular sites serve advice that denounces lifesaving vaccines and medications in an attempt to sell "alternative" remedies. And even the best websites often mix good data with pseudoscience so seamlessly that it's impossible to tell fact from fiction.

This information overload has made it impossible to sort through parenting guidance, let alone find a one-stop shop for reputable and realistic recommendations. When my daughter was born, I pieced together blog-based advice with my own expertise and scientific articles, but I never truly felt that I had a guidebook that I could trust. I wondered: Why isn't there a parenting book that not only presents a more balanced overview of the evidence, but also adds both the expertise of a pediatrician and the experience of a real-life millennial mother?

So I decided to write it. This book is a nuanced, beyond-the-basics parenting guide inspired by the very real questions I'm routinely asked—not just by my patients, but by friends feeling overwhelmed with the sheer amount of information available to them, and the frustration of trying to follow the rigid guidelines official pediatric organizations preach. Parenting is more complicated than ever, and I've spent years examining the evidence and integrating this data into my clinical and personal practice. As you read this book, you'll learn the reasoning and science behind official recommendations so that you can make smart decisions in concert with your pediatrician. I know how little evidence we have about many hot-button parenting topics, and I'm not afraid to admit when the experts are engaging in mere guesswork. But I'm not here to toss the baby with the proverbial stress-inducing guideline bathwater. Instead, this book will prove that good science and clinical insight are still important—but they only matter if they are translated into recommendations that are realistic and reasonable enough for you to follow.

Despite limitations in the field of pediatric medicine, I've been able to use the science and my own clinical expertise to create safe and realistic guidance. It's what I do every day. As a fully boarded pediatrician, my training includes four years of medical school, three years of pediatrics residency, plus continued daily work as a hospital pediatrician. Sorting through data, staying up-to-date on health and safety recommendations for kids, and knowing how to translate scientific evidence into clinical advice is literally my job.

This book is for everyone—and I mean everyone. It's no secret that most mainstream, "comprehensive" parenting tomes have a very specific view of what the default "traditional" family looks like. And while I'm delighted to share my advice with family and friends who look like me, my patients, and their families, all families across the country deserve to see themselves reflected in every corner of a comprehensive parenting guide. Universal guidance is only "universal" if it understands the challenges of those outside the "traditional" parenting setup. My goal is to show you that you can be amazing parents—even in the face of the unique challenges presented by our society's disparities and inequalities—no matter what your family looks like.

You'll probably notice some themes threaded through this book. The first is that while there is no one right way to parent, there are some safe and reasonable options that can guide decision-making. That's what I'm here to show you, and you'll see that in many cases, rigid schedules and rules are less effective than sound philosophy that you can adapt to your own lifestyle. You'll also learn that while a "guilt-free" approach is well-intentioned, you can't ignore science if you want to keep your baby—and yourself—healthy and safe. And above all, I'm here to show you why parental health *is* infant health. This book will teach you how to value your own health and happiness as much as your little one's, which, as luck will have it, benefits your baby too!

At the end of each chapter, you'll see key takeaway points, which are here for you during those frantic new parent moments when you need a quick refresher on what to do, or just a reminder on why you are doing just fine. These sections not only synthesize the most important information from each chapter, but they also give you a glimpse into the insights of my community of fellow pediatrician parents. My "5 out of 5 Pediatrician Parents Agree" seal of approval will let you know that pediatrician parents across the country echo and embrace my realistic, scientific, and compassionate advice.

Modern parenting comes with challenges that only a

modern parent can understand. As both a pediatrician and a mother, this is the book I wish I'd had when my daughter was born. While there may be no one way to raise your kids, there are still safe and realistic options that can guide you on your journey.

The internet may have broken parenting, but I'm here to fix it.

PART ONE

Birth to 3 Months

1

A NEWBORN SHOT
AND SOME EYE DROPS

• •

Vitamin K, Erythromycin,
and Other Medical Questions
to Worry about (or Not)
in Your Baby's First 48 Hours

My childbirth experience was certainly more dramatic than many. After a grueling eight months of a pregnancy plagued with hyperemesis (intense vomiting requiring IV fluids), I laughed that my due date couldn't come soon enough. My "wish" was granted when I was diagnosed with a low-lying placenta that required a scheduled early C-section. As the physical and emotional weight of pregnancy bore down on me into my third trimester, I joked that we should move up the delivery date even further. Lo and behold, at thirty-five weeks' gestation and still premature, my daughter complied. I sat at brunch on my only day off from an eighty-hour resident physician workweek and finished the last bite of my poached eggs mere minutes before I went into labor. I instantly realized the gravity of my situation: My placenta's position made it possible that I would lose blood quickly and dangerously. Over the next few hours, brunch turned into an emergency room visit turned into a swift trip to the operating room where my daughter was born. Happy birthday!

Needless to say, my birth experience was highly "medicalized." But even if I had been able to have a "natural" delivery, or at least a less unpredictable experience of labor and childbirth, I was fully prepared as a pediatrician (who had spent her fair share of time in the newborn nursery) for the first forty-eight hours in the hospital and what that meant for my baby. So before heading into the OR, I still remembered to tell my nurse that I wanted my daughter to get "everything," right after she came out.

There is so much planning, excitement, and preparation as we await the arrival of our little ones (raise your hand if your Pinterest board of nursery design inspiration was filled days after your first positive pregnancy test 🙋🏻‍♀️). So why do so many parents arrive in the delivery room unprepared for the barrage of medical decisions they will be asked to make for their newborn? It's not their fault! Somehow, during the months before parents meet their infants, few are told what to expect in the twenty-four to forty-eight hours after childbirth. Baby books often skip the period right after delivery, and pediatricians rarely have access to parents before their baby is born. Even the most prepared parents, with a library's worth of guidebooks in their baby bags, are frequently surprised and overwhelmed.

Until now. Let's review exactly what I meant when I eagerly agreed to my daughter getting "everything," and why I was so sure that this was a safe, necessary, and stress-free decision. I'm here to let you in on a trade secret that pediatricians wish wasn't such a secret: the official "Newborn Checklist." It's what pediatricians in the newborn nursery use to make sure you and your baby are ready to safely leave the hospital. It includes a bunch of shots, tests, and medicines that you'll be asked to opt into during your baby's first hours of life—all of which are safe and important. After I break down the science and rationale behind each intervention, I promise you will be fully prepared to say yes without an extra moment's thought. No need to face your baby's first medical decisions on the spot. Instead, it's time to take advantage of the wonders of modern medicine without any angst or doubt.

The Newborn Checklist

❏ Give the routine vitamin K injection that prevents serious bleeding (this can be done in the delivery room).

❏ Give antibiotic eye ointments to prevent the most common infections that cause newborn blindness (which can also be done right away in the delivery room).

❏ Give the hepatitis B immunization that will prevent your baby from ever getting this deadly virus. This is by far the most effective if given in the first days of a baby's life.

❏ Make sure that the baby doesn't lose too much weight, that their blood pressure, heart rate, and oxygen are okay, and that their physical examination is normal. Check that someone on the medical team has seen your baby feed at least twice, making sure they are swallowing well and getting enough milk.

❏ Make sure that your baby has peed and pooped at least once.

❏ Check jaundice level (called bilirubin) by placing a special flashlight on your baby's chest.

❏ Do a quick blood test (one drop of blood is taken from your baby's foot and placed onto a sheet of paper) that tests for dozens of genetic disorders that we would need to treat as quickly as possible to avoid serious and permanent damage. These include anemia from sickle cell disease, malnutrition and infections from cystic fibrosis, and brain and developmental problems from enzyme deficiencies like phenylketonuria.

❏ Do a quick newborn hearing test. A technician will bring a machine and adorable headphones to the room and will make sure that your baby's brain waves respond to sound. While it's important to check this box, hearing problems are rare. We just need to catch them early if they are there so we can address them as quickly as possible!

❏ Perform an extremely quick, easy, and noninvasive screening test for the major, serious newborn heart diseases by placing a sticker that measures your baby's blood oxygen level on their fingers and toes.

❏ Give some good old-fashioned counseling: Helping with breastfeeding, talking about safe sleep, making sure things are safe at home, reviewing car seat safety, and making sure that your baby can be seen by a pediatrician within a few days of leaving the hospital.

That's the quick and dirty, and it's totally okay to feel reassured by that brief overview and move on to the next chapter (I won't be offended). But if you have any lingering doubts, or just want to hear the juicy details of how and why these tests came to be, I've got you covered. Here's the deep-dive, scientific and expert reasoning behind each recommendation. Buckle up.

K Is for Kindness: Why the Vitamin K Injection Is Truly Great

Let's start with that routine vitamin K injection, which has become increasingly controversial—and with devastating consequences. In the bad old days, (i.e. before 1961 in the United States), one of the many scary things that could happen to a newborn was severe bleeding from a lack of vitamin K. Dietary vitamin K is an essential molecule that our livers use to make compounds that clot blood and stop serious bleeds. Vitamin K doesn't travel well across the placenta, making newborns susceptible to two different types of bleeding.

The first and most common, called "classical" vitamin K

deficiency bleeding (VKDB), occurs in the first week of life. The CDC estimates that as many as one in one hundred otherwise healthy newborns will experience this type of bleeding—usually at the umbilical cord or circumcision site—if they don't receive the routine Vitamin K injection. While this form tends to be milder, blood loss can still be severe, requiring urgent medical attention and admission to the hospital for monitoring and treatment (which is far more disruptive to bonding than a quick shot in the delivery room!). In fact, the only reason we view it as "mild" is because our medical care for newborn babies is so advanced. In other countries, babies still routinely die from this form: A study in Ethiopia in 2011 showed a 25% mortality rate for infants with classical vitamin K deficiency. It's hard enough to stay sane during those first few weeks at home, so adding the task of vigilantly monitoring your baby's skin for early signs of bleeding (when the consequences of missing it could not be higher) is a surefire—and unnecessary—way to add to new parent stress.

The second type of bleeding, "late" vitamin K deficiency bleeding, is the stuff of pediatrician and parent nightmares. It appears when a baby is between two and twelve weeks old, and is almost always life-threatening. This type is even harder to recognize, for doctors and parents alike, without the superficial bruising and bleeding that can sometimes help warn us that early VKDB is on the way. The earliest sign is usually just fussiness related to bleeding in the brain and/or belly. This means that any baby who missed their vitamin K shot and has an extra colicky day (which is most babies, since as luck would have it, two to twelve weeks is the exact same peak age for colic to emerge), will need to be seen in the emergency room. If the emotional toll of heading back to the hospital for an urgent brain ultrasound isn't enough, it gets even worse. Even with this timely evaluation and modern medical care, one out of every five babies with this condition will die, and many survivors suffer permanent injury. Unfortunately, once bleeding has started, giving vitamin K can't reverse any of it, and our best medicine is still damage control. A study from Vanderbilt University in 2014 found that 40% of late vitamin K deficiency bleeding survivors showed signs of serious brain dysfunction and disability.

This is not to alarm you. I only share this truly tragic and horrifying part of newborn medicine because it is something that you will have absolutely zero reason to worry about. Why? Because science outdid itself with this one. In 1944, Swedish researcher Jörgen Lehmann and his colleagues published their seminal study of over thirteen thousand infants who were given vitamin K at birth. The findings were revolutionary, showing a dramatic decrease in bleeding risk and cutting the rate of infant death by more than half. Shortly after, universal vitamin K administration became the standard of care, and it's been a hallmark of every hospital newborn checklist since. By the late twentieth century, late VKDB was declared eradicated altogether in the United States, a distant nightmare for American parents and pediatricians alike.

Makes vitamin K shots sound pretty amazing, right?

The short answer is simple: Yes, they *are* amazing. But parenting blogs and pseudomedical websites are filled with advice to the contrary, and well-meaning but misinformed parents are refusing vitamin K shots with alarming frequency. Those pediatricians at Vanderbilt University rekindled their love of vitamin K research in 2014 for a reason. In 2013, the hospital was thrust into the spotlight when six infants were diagnosed with late vitamin K deficiency bleeding. The results were tragic and predictable: Four of these babies had brain bleeding, two had bleeding in their intestines, and while all survived, two needed emergency brain surgery, at least one has serious brain damage (severe cognitive delays and complete right-sided paralysis), and two have moderate brain injuries.

It's not just Nashville. Vitamin K refusal has reached an all-time high nationally, and it's growing steadily. A national survey from the Better Outcomes through Research for Newborns (BORN, a network of clinicians in 34 states who treat 330,000 newborns) found that 52% of doctors and nurses now deal with vitamin K refusal. Numbers are even higher at non-hospital birthing centers that offer low-intervention care approaches. In these facilities, the refusal rate was recently shown to be 31%, over ten times higher than the refusal rate for in-hospital births.

What on earth happened? While it's important not to blame the online misinformation highway for all of society's woes, let's blame the internet (at least mostly) for this one. When Vanderbilt investigated why those six families had refused vitamin K, they found that misinformation was at the center of each one. A quick trip to Google reveals dozens of dangerous vitamin K lies. You'll hear that vitamin K causes cancer later in childhood (it doesn't); that the vitamin K injection traumatizes babies (it doesn't, and they just went through a way bigger trauma that they all get over, I promise); or, most commonly, injections are unnatural, unnecessary, unimportant. These claims have all been thoroughly debunked. The only "risks" of vitamin K injection are local pain, soreness, discomfort, and a theoretical but yet-to-be-seen risk of infection or injury to adjacent structures.

But misinformation has persisted and continues to spread. Parenting blogs, social media groups, and even less-reputable practitioners all frequently espouse anti-vitamin K falsehoods and hide the true dangers of vitamin K deficiency bleeding. Based on my experience with parents I've counseled and what I've seen online, it comes as no surprise to me that only one of the families in Nashville even knew that life-threatening bleeding was possible without the vitamin K injection.

Pediatricians don't counsel parents to say yes just because it's the status quo, but because we know it's what we need to do to keep infants healthy. I promise you that the benefits of vitamin K are enormous, that I was eager and excited for my daughter to get hers immediately after birth, and that you can and should ignore every piece of (often for-profit) misinformation.

I know what you're up against. I've seen this extremely compelling and extremely dangerous misinformation first-hand. I'll never forget when the parents of Ella, a newborn I cared for in the nursery right after she was born, told me they were refusing her vitamin K injection. I had just completed my physical examination (she was adorable and healthy), and as an exhausted resident it was so tempting to simply shrug, sigh, and hand a waiver for the parents to sign confirming that they accepted the risks of refusal. But as I swaddled this beautiful baby and placed her back in the arms of her clearly loving parents, I was overcome by a feeling I just couldn't shake. How could such good parents make such a bad decision?

I took off my gloves, put my pager aside (hello, residency in the year 2016!), and sat down with Ella's mother and father for an uninterrupted, face-to-face conversation. I knew this was an important moment, that they were excited and exhausted and just wanted to snuggle their new baby, but would they be willing to walk me through their thought process? Unsurprisingly, they had done extensive research, but relied on unverified, pseudoscientific sites for their information. Like one "mom blog" post that was convincing enough to give even me pause. While the blog's author acknowledged that she is "not a doctor" and denied giving medical advice, she ingeniously cherry-picked excerpts from legitimate studies to misrepresent data in a way that completely misunderstood science. One section detailed studies showing that mothers who eat a certain diet can make their breast milk rich with vitamin K, allowing the reader to assume that this will be enough to prevent vitamin K deficiency bleeding (it won't: formula-fed babies can have serious bleeding too, and that milk is fortified with vitamin K). Another paragraph offered maternal consumption of her own placenta as a quick vitamin K boost, without explaining that placenta-eating doesn't just give moms a nice dose of vitamins and minerals (still not enough to prevent VKDB), but also risks serious bacterial infections. She concluded that her approach—eschewing the lifesaving injection for vitamins and teas that she shills—was responsible, safe, and scientific (but remember, hundreds of commenters who thank her for arming them to refuse the vitamin K shot and buy her teas instead, this is not medical advice!).

It took me more than an hour to patiently detail the science and debunk the myths with Ella's parents, sharing real patient stories, and ultimately taking a strong stance: As a pediatrician (and now as a mother), I was and am 100% confident that routine vitamin K administration is the way to go.

Ella's parents ended up agreeing to her vitamin K injection, and I was delighted. But this turned out to be a rare case where I was able to change parents' minds. The reality is that pediatricians, myself included, don't routinely have the time to sit and undo all the damage done by online misinformation. And the results are tragic. Not statistics, not blog posts, not theoretical numbers. Real babies suffer, and real families are heartbroken. Like Teddy, a patient who suffered a serious brain bleed after missing his vitamin K shot and, despite emergency surgery, now lives with permanent brain damage and seizures even as a school-aged child. His parents, like so many others whose children suffered from vitamin K deficiency bleeding, wish they had been given the knowledge and recommendations needed to make the most informed and safest decisions.

If you're thinking: Whoa, I thought this chapter was supposed to *remove* the stress of the newborn period, not make me terrified of horrible things that could happen to my baby, I still got you! There's no need to worry for a single second about any of this once you shut out the noise, decide that vitamin K is a no-brainer, and go back to packing your hospital bag with as many comfy pajamas and contraband pacifiers (we'll get to that later) as you can fit in.

The Gift of Sight:
Erythromycin Eye Drops FTW

Another sometimes-controversial newborn rite of passage is an antibiotic eye ointment called erythromycin. Let's review a brief history before jumping into the latest (needlessly) hot-button discussion.

As early as the 1800s, doctors noticed a common and serious problem. At the time, one in ten babies born across Europe developed inflammation of their conjunctivae (the thin layer of tissue under your eyelids and over parts of the whites of your eyes) in the first few weeks of life. They called this "ophthalmia neonatorum," and as more research was done, it turned out that 3% of these babies went on to become blind. That means that three in one thousand babies born across the continent became permanently blind, for unclear reasons, and with no prevention or treatment.

In 1879, there was a breakthrough. Dr. Albert Neisser in Germany shared his finding that mothers with gonorrhea had babies with ophthalmia neonatorum. It made sense, since doctors had suspected that it was related to bacteria that passes from moms to babies through the birth canal. Just a year later, another German doctor, Carl Credé, decided to put silver nitrate (an antiseptic, but very irritating solution) in all babies' eyes when they were born, rather than waiting until they developed symptoms—at which point it almost never helped. It was wildly successful, with his hospital showing a thirtyfold reduction in ophthalmia neonatorum cases that year.

It's been 140 years since the initial discovery that eye drops can prevent blindness in babies. Obviously, things have changed. The world of infectious diseases is much more complicated, and a new organism called chlamydia has taken over gonorrhea as the most common sexually transmitted infection around the world (currently about six times more common than gonorrhea in women in the United States).

We also have antibiotics. We routinely screen people who are pregnant for sexually transmitted infections like gonorrhea and chlamydia, and we're able to give effective antibiotics to treat them during pregnancy. Ophthalmia neonatorum is therefore much, much less common than it used to be, especially in areas with access to prenatal care and the resources to follow through with testing and treatment. And when we do see ophthalmia neonatorum, we can give a baby antibiotics and almost always prevent blindness.

Why, then, do many countries with low rates of ophthalmia neonatorum, like the United States and Canada, still give all babies eye ointment to prevent it? As always, it's about comparing risks and benefits. The invention of antibiotics—and the continuous development of better antibiotic options—means that we haven't used silver nitrate for decades, which did cause serious chemical irritation and even temporary vision problems. We instead use 0.5% erythromycin, which does not cause any significant irritation and has no serious side effects *at all*. The only "risk" of giving eye drops to every single baby born is just the cost. Any time there is a universal screening or prevention measure, public health experts have to look closely at the numbers and decide if the benefits are worth the resources, time, and money. So when Australia and Great Britain decided to do away with their erythromycin-for-all newborn policy, I didn't think twice about its safety or efficacy for *my* baby. I knew it was just a boring financial decision.

I also had no qualms about erythromycin ointment even though I knew my daughter was at extremely, extremely low risk of getting an eye infection. I had routine prenatal testing and was quite confident that I didn't have gonorrhea or chlamydia. I may have had other bacteria like staphylococcus or streptococcus species, which now account for about one third of ophthalmia neonatorum cases and may also be prevented with erythromycin, but I was having a scheduled C-section. This meant that transmission of any badness that lived in my birth canal was incredibly unlikely (but not impossible, since bacteria can travel up into the womb, usually after your water breaks). Why on earth, then, would I agree to give my daughter something designed to prevent an infection she almost certainly did *not* have?

Because I wanted to protect my baby's eyesight. It was that simple. When I talk about comparing risks and benefits, or when others come at you with the data, the numbers, the relative rates of goodness or badness happening to your baby, it doesn't mean anything without context. Here's the context: There are no serious side effects from erythromycin ointment. None. I knew that at the time of delivery, a nurse would place a tiny bit of antibiotic goo in my baby's already goo-filled eye, that would sit like Vaseline (which is what it mostly is) on her eyeballs and not even get to her bloodstream. I also knew that it would prevent my baby from needing oral or intravenous antibiotics if she had any signs of possible eye infection. Most babies have clogged tear ducts or some viral eye goop early in life, and if they haven't been protected with erythromycin ointment, the safest thing is to give some just-in-case antibiotics that do have real side effects.

It's okay to refuse to overcomplicate things. Agonizing over the likelihood that you have an STI is an unnecessary intellectual exercise. When I decided to say yes to erythromycin ointment, I knew there was no need to reflect on my extremely strong marriage, view a public health measure as a personal attack on my relationship, or waste time parsing through the highly improbable but not impossible odds that I had an asymptomatic sexually transmitted disease or undetected skin bacteria. It would have mattered if there were any risks to this awesome preventive measure. But there really aren't. When we balance risk and benefit, we can't just think about the frequency of goodness or badness, we also have to consider the magnitude. Erythromycin ointment is like having a life vest on an airplane. Even though the odds of my needing a life vest during a crash, water landing, or other super-scary scenario are fortunately slim, you won't see me on a plane that doesn't have one ready for me if I need it. And just like having life vests on an aircraft isn't an attack on the pilot's skills, my wanting to preserve my baby's vision wasn't an attack on my sexual health. I chose her eyes over my pride and haven't looked back since.

Queen B: There Is Definitely No Need to Delay Baby's First Vaccine

After a more nuanced understanding of risk-and-benefit comparison courtesy of our erythromycin ointment discussion, I hope you'll be primed to embrace why saying yes to my daughter's first vaccine was a stress-free decision. The serious risks of this newborn shot are the same as the risks of a vitamin K injection: none. Later, in my vaccine chapter, you'll see how decades of rigorous research have proven, more than any other intervention known to modern medicine, that all recommended childhood vaccinations are safe and most effective in the current doses and with the current schedule. It's an uncomfortable poke, but again pales in comparison to the rite of passage your baby has just completed to get from their cozy uterine hot tub to the cold, outside world. And by doing it at the same time as the lifesaving vitamin K injection, it's a single and combined moment of discomfort.

But pediatricians, of course, don't recommend anything that doesn't have real benefit, even if the risks are zero. Hepatitis B is a devastating, deadly virus. Acute infection can be mild in babies and adults alike, but it can also cause life-threatening liver failure. Even scarier, nine out of ten newborns who get hepatitis B develop a *chronic infection*, which leads to liver failure or liver cancer—both frequently fatal—later in life.

Hepatitis B is spread mostly by blood, through sexual activity, and through the birth canal (which we call "vertical transmission"). For my daughter, just as with erythromycin, my prenatal testing and C-section delivery, alongside my own complete vaccine series and lack of high-risk behaviors, put her at extremely low risk of getting hepatitis B. But it wasn't zero. Prenatal lab tests are drawn early in pregnancy, leaving plenty of time for me to acquire hepatitis B, even if the chances were small. There have been case reports of transmission through saliva, through open cuts when people's skin touches, and as a hospital worker and someone out and about in the world, I wouldn't bet my daughter's liver on my own super-low-risk status.

And why would I when the vaccine has been shown to have such amazing effects? In 1982, when the vaccine was introduced in the United States, three hundred thousand people were infected with hepatitis each year, including twenty thousand children! By the year 2006, universal hepatitis B vaccine at birth decreased rates of vertical transmission by 98%. And it's this decrease in vertical transmission that keeps hepatitis B rates on the decline. Your baby's vaccination will keep their entire generation, and those to come, even safer from this painful and deadly disease.

I also knew that the hepatitis B vaccine is by far the most effective in preventing vertical transmission if given in the first twenty-four hours of life. I've talked to countless parents who hear that waiting until their baby's first pediatrician visit for their first vaccine is the way to go. It's a claim that's never made sense to me and seems to be perpetuated by anti-vaccine groups who perhaps hope that instilling vaccine hesitancy from day one of your baby's life will set the stage for further vaccine delays and refusals. That's my best guess, because there is absolutely no benefit to waiting (I repeat: Pairing that shot up with the vitamin K injection is a one-stop-shop for lifesaving, and very temporary, discomfort), and each hour's delay decreases its benefits significantly.

In the end, I knew there would be plenty of opportunity in the first year to stress over the risks and benefits of medicines for my daughter when some less black-and-white decisions presented themselves (I'm looking at you, antibiotics for mild, probably viral ear infections). But this is another seat belt, just like all other childhood vaccines. A moment's discomfort for a potential life saved, and both in fact with a long history of lobbying movements against them (no joke, there was a huge effort to downplay the amazingness of seat belt laws in the name of profit but under the guise of personal liberty). So don't torture yourself. The science speaks for itself, and there will be plenty of time to agonize over trickier risk-benefit ratios later.

Baby's First Checkup(s): Sorry to Keep Bothering You, but It's Actually Important

Why are we pediatricians so obsessed with prodding and poking your precious baby right after they're born? It can be frustrating to have so many interruptions during your first few days' snuggles. I definitely could have used a bit more R & R during those initial postpartum hours, but I knew that there was a bare minimum of examining and counseling that simply had to be done. This included checking my daughter's heart rate, blood pressure, and oxygen every few hours for a while, and having a complete physical examination by a pediatrician once some quality skin-to-skin was had.

These initial checks are especially important in looking for the increasingly rare but still serious bloodstream infections that some babies are born with. This sounds a lot scarier than it is, I promise, and it's exactly because decades of research have given pediatricians and obstetricians the tools to detect, prevent, and treat neonatal bacterial infections and turn these once common tragedies into a distant nightmare. But it does mean that some newborns who have abnormal vital signs, were exposed to bacteria around childbirth, or just aren't acting exactly the way we would expect, might get a little extra attention. This is usually just an additional day of monitoring in the hospital, but it could mean a few doses of just-in-case antibiotics as well (we'll talk about this in much more detail in Chapter 3). More likely than not, this won't be something you have to deal with. But if it is, as stressful as it may be, remember that it doesn't mean your little bundle of joy has a serious infection, or that they are actually "septic" (we're using the word "sepsis" here to describe what we're ruling out, not what we are treating). Your baby will still be ready for uninterrupted snuggles at home in no time.

Daily weights, keeping track of her diapers, and watching her breast and bottle feed also helped my daughter's doctors know she wasn't getting dehydrated. If your baby *is* showing signs of dehydration, it's absolutely not your fault. What it usually means is that we are failing you—usually by not helping enough with breastfeeding or not using supplemental formula when we should be. Our constant hydration checks and breastfeeding evaluations aren't because we don't trust you, but because we don't trust ourselves (which we'll go over in much more detail in Chapter 7).

Hospital stays after delivery are much shorter than they used to be, with most families now heading home on the second, third, or fourth day of their baby's life. There's less time to look for issues—like jaundice, dehydration, and breastfeeding problems—that can be dangerous if left unaddressed. It makes the first few days a little busier than many parents expect. This doesn't mean that bonding isn't important. Many hospitals are working in earnest to try to protect your first moments with your little one. You should feel empowered to ask for immediate skin-to-skin if it's not standard practice, even after a C-section (I did it!), as long as your baby doesn't require any prolonged, urgent medical attention. Your pediatricians will do their very best to examine your baby only when you're ready for it. Unless there's a medical problem, most pediatricians consider breastfeeding sessions, skin-to-skin with *any* parent, or even a family photo shoot to be reasons enough to wait on our full physical examination.

But at some point, at least once each day, your baby's doctor will need to check them out head-to-toe. Some examples of how daily checkups benefit your baby include:

1. Listening with our stethoscopes to find heart murmurs, some of which appear in the days following birth and can signal life-threatening problems.

2. Detecting anatomical variations like cleft lips and palates, which can cause serious feeding issues if not recognized early.

3. Picking up dimples and skin tags on baby's ears that clue us into kidney problems in some babies (I know, it's crazy!).

4. Looking for dimples, hair, and birthmarks on baby's backs that tell us to check out a baby's spinal cord.

It's important to be prepared not only for those frequent interruptions, but also for the possibility that your baby will have one of those physical examination findings that requires further workup. Please remember: As with all the screening tests, the majority of these variations are *not* a problem. Most murmurs, dimples, ear tags, and birthmarks are absolutely nothing to worry about. It's just important to figure that out sooner, and an extra ultrasound of the heart or spine is an extremely low-risk way to make sure we're not missing anything.

Diaper Duty: Please Be Patient and Wait for Those First Wet and Dirty Diapers

This is one of the less controversial items on the Newborn Checklist, but I want to make sure you're prepared for every box your baby will need to check before heading out of the hospital for in-home snuggles. Most babies will have a wet and dirty diaper in the first few days of life, and this doesn't often hold up discharge. But when it does, it's for good reason: It's crucial to make sure that a brand-new baby has peed and pooped because this lets pediatricians know that their urinary and gastrointestinal systems are healthy. There are certain anatomical issues in how a baby's kidneys, bladder, intestines, and other connective tubing form that are both totally serious and totally fixable. As with most newborn conditions, it's all about timing. If we detect these problems in the first few days, we can fix them and avoid scary and long-term consequences. Some babies take a little longer than others to get things going, so try not to stress if you have to stay in the hospital an extra day or two to prove your little one's plumbing is in working order.

#bilibaby: How a Flashlight Can Actually Keep Your Baby Out of the Hospital

While the science of newborn jaundice (yellow or ruddy-red skin at birth) is constantly evolving and quite complicated, what you need to know as a new parent is simple. Jaundice happens when a baby's body has a high level of something called "bilirubin," which is a substance the body creates naturally when it breaks down red blood cells. For most newborns, this is because their cute little livers aren't developed yet, so they have trouble converting bilirubin into the form that their body can pee or poop out. There are very, very rare cases where this high level of bilirubin can cause serious brain problems. If your baby's skin is glowing yellow, orange, or deep red, they might get a poke on their heel to check their bilirubin level in the lab. If not, they'll likely just have a flashlight placed on their chest that gives doctors a good guess of the possible range of their bilirubin level. If it's high enough, we'll confirm with that quick heel poke.

If the bilirubin level is above a certain threshold (which changes based on how many hours old your baby is, if your baby was born early, or if there are any other medical issues going on), your baby will get "phototherapy." I went through this with my daughter and know how upsetting it is to hear that your baby needs medical treatment, even if it is in fact just lying under warm purple lights in an Isolette. Most babies won't need more than the quick flashlight test, but even if they do need phototherapy, it almost never means there's any serious or long-term problem, and their stressful spa day under the glowing lights will soon be but a distant memory.

The Incredible, Phenomenal, Lifesaving, Science-Affirming Newborn Screen

There's one more quick poke, but this one is a blood test. Your baby's medical team will get one drop of blood from their heel and place it on a sheet of paper. This one drop of blood has saved lives across the nation, led to long and happy childhoods, and prevented so much devastation that it is hard to overstate just how much of a miracle the "newborn screen" really is.

While some diseases that we look for will be different depending on which state your baby is born in, most are the same. All of them are genetic conditions that, if found in the first days of life, can be treated in a way that either saves an infant's life entirely, or has such a meaningful impact on their health that waiting even one day more to find it would have horrible consequences. Some examples of the serious, life-threatening consequences that can develop without this early detection include anemia from sickle cell disease, malnutrition and infections from cystic fibrosis, and brain damage and death from enzyme deficiencies like phenylketonuria (PKU). I've personally seen babies whose lives were literally saved when diseases like PKU, congenital adrenal hypoplasia, and severe combined immunodeficiency were detected and treated right away. I've also seen cases where early screening wasn't done and cases were missed, truly preventable tragedies that I hope to never have to see again.

31

Can You Hear Me Now?: Get Ready for the Cutest Headphones You'll Ever See

Here's another low stress item that provides for a great photo-op (go google "newborn hearing screen" and tell me those tiny headphones aren't simply adorable). A specialized technician will bring a machine and newborn-sized headphones to the room and make sure that baby's brain waves respond to sound. There are a good number of false positives, mostly because newborns, it turns out, aren't the most cooperative patients. You may see that your baby "failed" one or both ears in their hearing screen. This is by far most commonly due to the fact that your incredible bundle of joy was simply not feeling it, and the data was insufficient. So don't stress and just bring your newborn back for a repeat test when they're a little older (you'll be given a follow-up plan before discharge). They'll likely pass with flying colors.

Can a Sticker Really Prevent Sudden Death in Newborns? (Spoiler Alert: Yes It Can.)

In fancy medical speak, we call this one the critical congenital heart disease (CCHD) screen. This test is one of the least invasive (it's literally placing a sticker on your baby's fingers and toes), but it saves thousands of lives each year. In the United States, about 7,200 babies are born with a type of heart condition that we describe as critical congenital heart disease. This means that without early medicines and even emergency surgery, a baby won't get enough oxygen to their body and can die suddenly in the first few days of life. But don't worry! The CCHD test is extremely good at picking up these terrifying heart problems. It's why pediatricians are *obsessed* with this one, and you should be too. By measuring the level of oxygen in the blood on different limbs, we can find the majority of these scary situations before babies even leave the hospital, and get them the lifesaving treatment they need. Wild, right? Science is so cool.

Here to Help: You'll Get a LOT of Guidance, but Don't Worry about Remembering It All

Pediatricians are nosy, but it's for good reason. If you are welcoming your little one into your family through birth, this is the first time that you and your baby aren't essentially the same patient. Your OB and/or midwife team has been doing an amazing job of looking out for both of you. But now it's our turn! We want to jump in and help take care of you both, focusing on your baby's medical issues while also embracing that the best way for your baby to be healthy is for their parents and all caretakers to be as happy and healthy as possible. You'll have to endure some personal questions and advice on breastfeeding, sleep, home safety, getting car seats and transportation ready, and setting up a pediatrician appointment. No need to memorize or take notes, though. You should get plenty of handouts, and your pediatrician is available day and night to answer any questions that arise.

If this isn't your first rodeo and there's an older sibling at home waiting to meet your next bundle of joy, a seasoned pediatrician is likely to share a few pro-tips on how to help welcome your new addition. It will be a time of transition—with plenty of older sibling emotions, behavioral changes, and a good dose of stress for the whole family—no matter what. But there are ways to make it less painful for everyone. The pediatrician parents I know generally favor trying to meet the new baby at home, not at the hospital, so that your older child will feel more comfortable, see you in a familiar setting, and have a bit of a "home field" advantage. We also are big fans of having a small gift "from the new baby" on hand and having one parent go inside first without baby to greet and prepare.

Jealousy is inevitable, but strategies that put an older sibling's needs first when it's so easy for them to become deprioritized with a much needier, more fragile baby, go a long way. Newborn and toddler crying at the same time? Go to the toddler first. If the newborn is in a safe place, they'll be okay to cry for a few minutes, and big sib will feel cared for, remembered, and protected, knowing that you are able to respond just as quickly as before a tiny intruder came to compete for their parent's attention. And all kids and adults—and especially toddlers—do best hearing "yes" instead of "no." Thinking ahead for some age-appropriate expressions of love and helpful tasks for your older child (handing you wipes for diaper changes, caring for their own doll or stuffed animal in parallel, giving the baby kisses on their toe rather than face) will help diffuse the inevitable tension.

There's an increasing, understandable frustration with how medicalized the birthing and postpartum experiences have become. More than likely, you'll hear people espouse the virtue of having "nature run its course" and encouraging you to decline incredible newborn preventive medical miracles. I understand, I promise. As a new mom, I was exhausted by the poking and prodding my daughter went through in those first days after she was born. But as a doctor, I knew that each specific intervention was carefully designed to keep my baby safe—and even save her life. Newborns are fragile, and infant morbidity and mortality are the real consequences of saying no to any newborn checklist item. So while I absolutely struggled with my own birth trauma and medicalized recovery, I wouldn't have completed our newborn checklist any differently.

I promise there will be situations where the "natural" route makes sense, or where a nontraditional approach to infant care is a reasonable, safe option. But those first few days of your baby's life don't leave a lot of room for error. Reimagining the newborn recovery period, optimizing your bonding, and pushing our hospital systems to create the best possible birthing experience are complex tasks. Removing lifesaving interventions in an attempt to achieve these goals, however, is misguided and can have devastating consequences. I give you permission to trust in good science and let the pediatricians at the bedside do what decades of lifesaving science have proven newborns need to survive and thrive. The Newborn Checklist, in the end, is just another part of being a loving, safe parent right from the very first day.

THE BOTTOM LINE

5 out of 5 Pediatrician Parents Agree

- The first forty-eight hours after your baby is born are filled with tests and treatments that keep them safe. Knowing what these are will help you feel relaxed and guarantee there are no surprises.

- It's safe to say yes to all of them without giving it a second thought. And yes, I mean all of them.

- The internet has a lot of scary information for why the vitamin K injection is dangerous—but it's not. Specifically, it will not traumatize a baby, can't cause cancer, and isn't "toxic" or "unnatural."

- The vitamin K shot (like all the items on the Newborn Checklist) is worth getting! Babies really do get sick (and even die) if we don't follow all these guidelines.

- The same is true for the other "controversial" items like erythromycin and the hep B vaccine. The benefits tower over any discomfort, there are no health risks, and providing this protection to your baby is the best way to be a safe and loving parent from the very first day of their life.

- Pediatricians want to partner with you to make your postpartum nesting period as calm and comfortable as possible. But there is a limit to how "natural" or "de-medicalized" your experience can be without sacrificing safety! Babies are fragile, and if nature had its way, we would have so many tragic outcomes. It's okay to just say yes to the preventive care that keeps you and your baby alive and well without overthinking it.

2

SWINGERS, ROCKERS, BOUNCERS, OH MY!

••

What You Need to Know about
Baby Products That Hold Your Infant
When You Can't

I remember the first time, before I had my own baby, that a
patient's parents asked me about baby gear. I had just finished performing my physical examination on Sophie, an
adorable and healthy two-week-old girl, and now it was time
for questions. I was only in my first months of training, but I
was eager to flex my clinical knowledge and share my advice.
Except instead of asking me about fevers, safe sleep, or developmental milestones, Sophie's parents wanted to know what I
thought about the Rock 'n Play, and did I have a baby swing
I could recommend? And while we were on the topic, at what
age should their baby start using the infant lounger? Was it
okay to place her in a Bumbo chair before she could sit on
her own? Also, should the portable bassinet be placed in the
Pack 'n Play or did that go straight onto the floor? Oh, and she

really loves being in the BabyBjörn but couldn't that cause a problem with her hips? Thanks, Doc.

I've never had a particularly good poker face, but I did my best to maintain some facade of doctorly confidence, sidestepping a real answer as I backed slowly out of the room. When I brought in my supervising doctor, she patiently reviewed her recommendations about each product in question, relying heavily on her years not only as a pediatrician but also as a mother of three young children. I sat in awe.

Over the following years of residency, I read the official American Academy of Pediatrics guidelines on the limited number of baby carriers they review. I memorized the AAP doctrine. Those seemingly cute baby walkers? Extremely dangerous and simply verboten. Orthopedic surgeons still think BabyBjörns are bad for hip development, but the data is shaky, and pediatricians agree that any possible risks pale in comparison to the real, enormous benefits of baby wearing. And unless there is a safety recall, and as long as parents are using rockers, bouncers, swings, and loungers according to the written safety instructions, pediatricians generally stay out of the product placement game.

When it was time to make my own registry years later, I thought it would be a piece of cake. I was, after all, a baby expert by trade. But as I clicked through a sea of Graco, Chicco, Fisher-Price, Boppy, UPPAbaby and Britax, my head swirled. Per my registry, I needed to add one of each type of carrier to the list and would get a free gift when I had done so! I was well into my second trimester, working eighty-hour weeks, and barely sleeping, so my brain had no space for consumer skepticism. I was a prime target for this marketing ploy.

My work was cyclical. First, I would finalize my list, with each bouncer, lounger, rocker, and swing chosen based on careful research and customer reviews. But then—did I hear about the latest car seat recall? I gasped, deleted, started over. Or my coworker would casually mention her amazing experience with the highest-end bassinet, which was only $150 more expensive than what I currently had on my registry. Of course I knew the rules of safe sleep and had read the Consumer Reports, and my existing bassinet was certainly up to snuff, but didn't it make sense for my daughter to get the best rest possible? I laughed, imagining taking my newborn daughter mattress shopping at the fictional bassinet section of a department store. "Baby, what do you think of the lower back support on this one? Should we try one with adjustable firmness and head elevation?" It was silly, an unnecessary cost and stress. But the next day, I added the expensive bassinet to my registry. Just in case.

When my daughter arrived, suffice to say we had way more gear than we needed. And after I talked myself out of the luxury brands, I was delighted by how well my "economy" items worked. My daughter seemed to prefer them.

There are endless products to hold infants during play and rest, and chances are, by the time you read this chapter, you've already added one of each to your baby registry. That's truly great if that's your shopping style! I'm not here to judge your spending practices, because getting ready for your little one means getting ready to part with a good chunk of your disposable income. Yet the reality is that for many parents, stocking up on baby gear has become more stressful than enjoyable. The possibilities are overwhelming, even for a pediatrician (me—I was overwhelmed!). Take away the pediatric training and add parenting blogs (even the best of which earn money by commissions when linked items are purchased), product recalls, competing registry advertisements, and good old-fashioned word-of-mouth fearmongering, and it seems impossible to sort through it all.

If you're reading this book, you're already a thoughtful, loving parent who only wants the best, safest products for your baby. When nearly every item on the booming baby market claims to hold this title, it becomes hard not to feel that spending your very last dollar on baby products is the only way to assure a lifetime of health and happiness. Before you dive in too deeply with your wish lists and purchases, let's examine which products are most useful—and, of course, pediatrician and parent approved. Here's my approach to navigating the online ocean of baby products. Sit back, relax, and use this framework to decide which baby holders are right for you. You'll feel all the joys of retail therapy with zero percent of the manipulative, guilt-inducing, anxiety-provoking consumer angst. Win-win!

Cost Matters—Just Not How You Think

First, let's dispel the most common myth: While splurging on a luxury item can get you improved portability, design, and aesthetics, dollar signs don't translate into safety. Think of purchasing baby holders more like shoe shopping than car shopping. For example, when I bought my Subaru (#basicpride), I spent all the money I had to make sure every single safety feature was on deck—fancy backup detector, lane departure, blind-spot, auto-braking, collision-prevention, you name it. Higher price tag, safer car. Not so with baby holders. Baby product manufacturers fortunately aren't allowed to commoditize safety, and there are basic standards they must meet for any reputable vendor to feel comfortable selling their products. Once a carrier has earned its seal of approval from Consumer Reports (consumerreports.org) or any similar, trusted safety organization, it's just as safe as the premium models. Of course, vendors may still sell certain types of products—in-bed sleepers, crib bumpers, and baby walkers, to name a few—that pediatrians disapprove of altogether (I'll go through these in their own special subsection, don't you worry). But price-comparison is irrelevant in these cases, since high-ticket items in this category are just as unsafe as their discount counterparts.

If that's the case, why are so many luxury baby holders wildly expensive? It's mostly a marketing game. The most dramatic price discrepancies are due to mere name recognition: A fancy brand-name stroller system with all the bells and whistles can easily run $900, compared to its equally safe but decidedly less-sexy standard-issue $200 counterpart. Besides brand allegiance and representation of higher status, the only other reason to spend more on these products is convenience, style, and preference. So while baby product shopping isn't like car shopping, it's a whole lot like shoe shopping. Once I realized that I couldn't spend all my money on the baby-carrier equivalent of the Subaru Eyesight safety pack-age that would save my daughter's life, I was able to make my registry exactly like I did my Zappos.com wish list.

Adding items to your registry should reflect how you and your family navigate comfort, aesthetics, cost, and brand rec-ognition. Are you the type of person who loves designer items and splurges on big names with your hard-earned money? Rock on! A $450 high-end travel crib is just for you. Do you live in a walk-up apartment, or think you'll need to use your stroller for commuting? You should probably prioritize por-tability, just like you would good arch support in your favor-ite pair of boots. Customer reviews can be overwhelming, and there are more listicles than I can count that promise to help you find the single perfect baby holder for every possible specification and personal preference. Grab your coffee, take your time to browse, but set some limits to your research. Decide on a few important attributes to focus on (may I sug-gest portability and ease of storage for the urban parent?), choose only a few review websites to give you options, and spend only as much extra time and energy comparing and browsing as brings you joy.

And if all else fails, just remember: It's hard to go wrong as long as basic safety standards have been met. In general, these products come in price ranges, just like a good pair of heels. The thirty-dollar stroller is not going to be as cute or portable as a mid-level model, but it will still be safe. And the mid-level model will lack some high-end convenience fea-tures, but it should otherwise stack up comparably in most situations. If, like me, you are willing to spend all the money on safety and comfort and zero money on labels (Real quote from me to car salesperson: "I would like your safest, ugliest car, please"), then your mid-range Graco/Chicco/Evenflo gear will be more than fine.

Take Your Time; There Will Always Be an Opportunity to Spend More Money Later

Registry checklists (with nominal "completion gifts" that often have a total value less than the cost of a basic onesie), social media pressure, and general expectant-parent panic all make it easy to think that you need to get everything now, all at once, before the baby has even arrived. Not so. Once you've figured out and embraced your baby-product style, you can ignore your registry's categories and resist the temptation to "complete" its checklist. I certainly did not succeed at this. Learn from my mistake: The money saved from passing on even one unnecessary item will buy you a dozen free-gifts-worth of diapers and wipes that you will desperately need.

There are essentially only three categories to baby holders: (1) Items that are good to have before the baby gets there; (2) Items you'll probably need (or at least want) later; and (3) Items that are so hit-or-miss with parents that you might not want them at all.

1. **Items that are good to have before the baby gets there**

    It's fine to start out with a place for safe sleep (likely a bassinet, but a Pack 'n Play is safe too, cheaper, and can be used for travel), a baby carrier, a car seat, a stroller, and . . . that's about it. No, really.

Besides diapers, wipes, pacifiers, and a few gallons of coffee per day (at least in my case), there isn't a whole lot of gear that's needed in those first few weeks at home. This makes more sense once you have an idea of what those first few weeks will be like. Newborns want to be almost constantly held for at least the first few weeks—a sleep-deprived reality that means you and whoever is around to help you will be playing a lot of pass-the-baby. ("No, it's my turn to shower"; "Just let her cry in the bassinet, I'll be there in a minute.") When your baby isn't being held, fed, or rocked, they'll hopefully be sleeping. We'll take a deep dive into safe sleep in Chapter 6, but the only places you'll be placing your newborn to sleep is in a crib, Pack 'n Play, or bassinet (or sometimes your own firm mattress, but we'll go into that later). Most parents choose some sort of bassinet (sometimes confusingly marketed as "co-sleepers" because they let your baby sleep *next* to your bed, not in it). It's rare to use your baby's crib for at least a few weeks (often a few months!), so feel free to take your time to get that nursery aesthetic just right and choose the crib of your design dreams.

The only other must-have baby holders for newborns are whatever you need for travel. This usually includes some sort of baby wearing device, which is useful not only for your trips out into the brave new world, but also for increased mobility around the house. Depending on how you travel, you may or may not need a car seat. I think it's always good to have, since taxis, Ubers, Lyfts, planes, and buses are safest with babies properly secured and strapped in. And of course, even the most in-shape parents need a stroller for longer journeys, leisurely strolls, or—God bless them—family jogs during parental leave.

TRANSLATION PLEASE!

WHAT ARE THESE CALLED ON MY REGISTRY?

Look for words and phrases like: bassinet, portable crib, travel crib, mini crib, Pack 'n Play, play yard, nursery center, bedside sleeper, co-sleeper (this is NOT an in-bed sleeper and must be the kind that has a firm mattress and is placed next to your bed, as we'll go over in Chapter 6), stroller, jogger, car seat, travel system, baby carrier, and baby wrap.

---

2. **Items you'll probably want later**

Many baby products fall into this second category, meaning you might want to wait to buy them until you have time to see what it's like to have a human baby at home. Does your little one like being rocked or bounced? That should help you decide if a bouncer or swing makes more sense. Infant loungers—which are just fancy baby pillows—are great, but remember, for the first few weeks, caretakers will almost always be holding their baby when they aren't safely sleeping in their bassinet.

Stressed at the idea of waiting until the crazy postpartum period to do more baby-product shopping? Looking to get everything on your registry right away so everyone knows what you need? Both? Me too! I'm the kind of planner who makes lists of the lists I'm going to make, so waiting until after my baby was born to get our gear was not even something I considered. And good thing, because I ended up being beyond overwhelmed with my postpartum struggles, both typical and extreme, and my family and I did not have one extra minute or ounce of energy to spend on registry shopping.

So in hindsight, even though we had much, much more gear than we needed, I would still have registered for everything I did with very few changes. I just would have held off on opening and assembling most of it. So many items were shoved in the closet, barely used or left unused entirely. For me, this included a fancy swing, since my daughter screamed every time we put her in her high-end $250 swing and could only be soothed by bouncing. Adding insult to injury, she would only stop crying when we picked her up and placed her in her $50 bouncer. It would have been nice to have some packages ready to exchange or return once the dust settled, so we could pocket that sweet cash or store credit for—you guessed it—a never-ending supply of diapers, wipes, and coffee.

TRANSLATION PLEASE!

WHAT ARE THESE CALLED ON MY REGISTRY?

Look for words and phrases like: infant lounger, newborn lounger, swing, bouncer, bouncing seat, rocking seat, and rocker.

---

3. There's a reasonable chance you'll never use any of these

The last category is the one that leads to the biggest loss of money (and sanity): Items that some parents and babies love, but many never really get into. Most of the items that are decidedly hit-or-miss are, conveniently, also the ones that babies don't use until they're at least a few months old. Since your baby won't be able to sit, even with support, until she is at least three to four months old, you'll have time to figure out if she's more of an ExerSaucer or jumperoo type of kid. Same for your foray into family meals, another seated activity. When we started solids at six months, we found that our daughter much preferred her $40 on-the-floor feeding seat to the $200 high chair we had been gifted. It was easier to clean, portable for picnics, and when we moved from Michigan to a smaller apartment in New York, we simply gave the high-end high chair away, almost completely unused.

Play mats, baby gyms, and other similar tummy-time setups will also go unused for many weeks, so take your time deciding on these as well. Yes, as a natural-born-planner, I would have still registered for many of these. But it would have been nice to shove those out of sight and out of mind into the darkest recesses of our home and wait to open them (or return them) until I'd had the chance to get a better sense of what my daughter clearly did and did not like.

TRANSLATION PLEASE!

WHAT ARE THESE CALLED ON MY REGISTRY?

Look for words and phrases like: high chair, booster seat, floor seat, feeding seat, Exer-Saucer, play gym, jumper, activity center, play mat, baby gym, jumperoo, and activity seat.

In the end, it's important to take a step back and remember that registries, blogs, websites, and social media are all selling something. And while it should go without saying, they've never been into your home or lived a day in your life! How could they know how many rooms need a baby-sized container, or which comfy couches lull you to sleep and need a safe sleep setup within arm's reach? I personally loved using my three-dollar plastic laundry basket instead of a second bassinet when I napped on the couch (and, of course, my cost-conscious daughter seemed to prefer it too.) But plenty of parents have multiple iterations of the same exact bassinet, travel crib, bouncer, swing, or rocker stationed in different nooks and crannies to assure they can easily and safely put their baby down in any room and at any time. Do what works for you! Use this purchasing timeline only as it serves you and your shopping needs, and you'll be fully prepared—not overprepared—for your little one's arrival.

Safety Is Simple—Once You Know What to Look For

While safety doesn't align with cost in the world of baby holders, there's still a way to ensure you're choosing the safest products possible. The first is to avoid the types of baby holders that pediatricians point-blank justifiably discourage. There are only a few product types that are verboten, so you can quickly cross these items off your list and move on to more exciting baby planning. Some baby beds adhere to safe sleep rules and some don't. Bassinets, cribs, and Pack 'n Plays are all great examples of the firm, flat, cushion-free items that conform to the evidence-based recommendations we have to assure babies sleep safely. Those DockATots, quilted bassinets, crib bumpers, and foldable travel cribs all don't. So keep it simple: don't buy them.

Most other products are fair game as long as they've met safety testing standards. The major category that comes up later in your baby's life is infant walkers. Pediatricians understandably shy away from recommending any of those adorable but legitimately dangerous baby walkers. Baby walkers give your little one zero developmental advantage and have been proven to have no benefit in helping babies learn to walk. What they instead allow is for infants to move more quickly and to more dangerous places than they would unassisted. This is why, even under supervision, thousands of babies take a trip to the emergency room from serious walker-related injuries. The most common accident is falling down stairs, but I've seen babies who knocked hot coffee off the table and suffered serious burns, and there have even been drowning or fall-related deaths. Yikes!

Again, there's no need to stress one bit. Just remove walkers with rollers, wheels, or other mobility enhancing attachments from your registry. When we got one as a very sweet and well-intentioned gift, we found that we could remove the wheels to turn it into a stationary activity center. And if that hadn't been an option, we would have graciously and gratefully exchanged it for an upright accessory that came free of accident-enhancing mobility our baby wasn't quite ready for.

TRANSLATION PLEASE!

WHAT ARE THESE CALLED ON MY REGISTRY?

You can just say no to anything that includes words or phrases like: infant sleeper, DockA-Tot, in-bed sleeper, crib bumper, quilted crib, and walker.

Once you've moved on from the unsafe baby product categories, there's no need to indulge in independent online safety research. Any brand at any price point—from an eighty-dollar Pack 'n Play to a five-hundred-dollar travel crib—that carries a Consumer Reports seal of approval, like those from consumerreports.org or jmpa.org—is equally safe. These sites have comprehensive lists of the items they feel pass safety standards, and these standards are high—if anything, so rigorous that some probably safe products don't make the cut. In addition, by registering your products, you'll be able to get updated information about recalls. Companies are very good about getting in touch with parents (just think of the PR nightmare if they don't) so trusting in warranties is totally safe and will remove the temptation to prowl the parenting blogs for terrifying and unnecessary alerts.

Finally, a quick injection of some much-needed common sense. A product is only as safe as how it's used, and as long as you use products as intended, your baby will be fine. It seems intuitive, but the newborn period is filled with so much worry that it's impossible to see the huge, all-caps warnings about suffocation that are plastered onto even the safest products and not feel a visceral jolt of panic. It's what I felt, and what my patient Frankie's mom disclosed to me at his one-month checkup. She was following safe sleep to the letter of the law and only allowed unsupervised sleep in the bassinet or empty crib. She used the infant lounger pillow when she was playing with Frankie on the floor, so why was it covered with INFANT DEATH RISK tags on every surface, seemingly intent on reminding her of her biggest postpartum fears?

The last thing Frankie's mom needed was a constant trigger for her anxiety. We made a plan, and I told Frankie's mom to place colored stickers over all the labels (cutting or marking out warnings makes them ineligible for warranty, or we would have gone that route). Out of sight, out of mind, but not in a way that negated safety—I was confident that Frankie's mom knew how this product should be used. If anything, I've found those warnings to be counterproductive or even tragically dangerous, creating warning label fatigue. To put it bluntly, it seems that every item on the market has a disclaimer—usually with scary labels right on the product—on how this safety-tested product could kill your baby. Focusing on common-sense rules for how to use baby products (those Consumer Reports sites provide a great framework) is the only way to preserve safety and sanity.

THE BOTTOM LINE

5 out of 5 Pediatrician Parents Agree

- Any baby holder that is blessed by the Consumer Reports safety seal is safe, so spending more on luxury items doesn't mean that a product is safer.

- There's no need to do independent safety research online from blogs and other websites, as long as it has a seal of approval from consumerreports.org or jmpa.org.

- These products are only as safe as how they are used; follow pediatrician guidelines to avoid the types of items we don't like in general.

- It's okay to spend more for comfort and aesthetics—it's just a personal preference, so don't let the other moms, dads, and product-shilling blogs bully you!

- Start with the essentials; there's always time to buy more gear later, and you'll want some time to see which types of products work best for you (spend that extra money on diapers and lattes!).

- Read the warning labels once and chat with your pediatrician to make sure you're using a product correctly. Then forget about them after that.

3

CRANK THE AC AND GET YOUR BOOSTERS

•••

The Rules for Bringing Your Newborn Outside and Welcoming Visitors

As a new parent, there's nothing more magical than snuggling at home all warm, cozy, and safe with your beautiful new baby. But even the most devoted parents are human, and people simply aren't designed to sit inside all day. All too often, new parents feel that the only way to assure their little one's health is to come down with a self-induced case of cabin fever. Not the case! In fact, I know personally, professionally, and scientifically that losing your last shred of parental sanity cooped inside is riskier than a well-planned field trip or play-date. So why is there so little tangible advice on how to balance getting out of the house, traveling, and having visitors with the risk of tiny newborns getting sick? Even before pandemic parenting and the age of quarantine-and-chill, it seemed impossible to find concrete, pediatrician-approved answers to parents' burning questions on newborn visitors and travel.

We can cut pediatricians a little slack with this one.

Since it's hard to study newborns, especially once they are out of the hospital, the science is limited. Without rigorous research, the American Academy of Pediatrics has yet to set forth guidelines, so many pediatricians understandably leave everything (mostly) up to parental discretion. But I know how complicated these decisions are, and how overwhelming it can be to feel like your tiny, precious baby's health lies solely in your hands.

It doesn't. While there is still room for discretion and individualized risk-benefit analysis (remember in Chapter 1 when I told you there'd be plenty of chances for nuanced decision-making?), you're not alone. I've found enough good research (and used plenty of common sense) to create a winning approach. It's what I used for my own postpartum planning and have been sharing with patient families and friends ever since.

As you may have already guessed, my new-parent worries were more intense than many. Working as a pediatrician in a busy hospital makes serious baby diseases seem way more common than they are. So when it came to the topic of venturing outside into the Michigan winter with my daughter, my thoughts roamed far beyond cute coats and mittens. Because she was tiny and premature, I knew she wouldn't be able to easily maintain her body temperature. And if she became too cold, she might need to go to the hospital to get warm. And if she went to the hospital to get warm, they would likely need to do a lot of tests to make sure that her temperature problems weren't because she had a serious bacterial infection. And if they did this, she would likely need to stay over in the hospital for a few nights to get antibiotics and wait for test results. Pregnancy and delivery had not been fun—the last thing I needed was a trip back to the hospital and more poking and prodding on my beautiful, exhausting new baby.

Having a new baby is already rough, so when you add on -10°F weather, a family that lives a plane ride away, and a husband who has to get back to work before you know it, you start to go a little crazy. Or at least I did. After a few weeks, it was time to make a plan. When would I leave the house? Where would I go? Who could come over? After much research and reflection on my clinical experiences, I was able to create a guide that balanced getting out of the house, traveling, and having visitors with the risk of tiny newborns getting sick—and that can still be applied to the challenging decision-making we all face in this post-covid world.

Knock, Knock: Can I Come In? (When to Let People Visit Your Tiny Bundle of Joy)

First, let's talk about why hosting visitors is even risky at all. There's only one major risk, which is exposure to germs. A new baby's immature lungs and underdeveloped immune system place them at a much higher risk of having bad infections of the blood and brain than older kids or adults.

There are two main flavors of bad baby germs: viruses and bacteria. With viral infections, including but definitely not limited to covid, newborns can have mild cold symptoms like anyone else, but more serious problems are also common—meaning that congested newborns can find themselves in the hospital with face masks, oxygen and breathing tubes, while their parents simply have a sore throat and sniffles. There's no medicine that babies need for viruses, and they will recover on their own, but it is possible that they'll need a lot more help getting there than you or I will.

The other danger of a cold virus is that even if a baby has mild symptoms, they will frequently have a fever as well; kids in general get higher fevers than adults, and babies are no exception. Fevers themselves aren't dangerous, but they can signal something dangerous: bacterial infections. And while older kids and adults have terrible pain, get confused, or have other symptoms that let doctors know their infection is probably big, bad, and bacterial, a newborn with a bacterial blood infection might show a fever—and that's it. Or be a little more tired than usual (almost impossible to detect in a newborn who sleeps twenty hours each day). Or not be awesome at feeding (just like many healthy new babies). So while most newborn fevers are harmless, a small number of them signal a serious problem that requires urgent medical attention.

Don't panic! Pediatricians are committed to making sure we don't miss a single serious newborn infection, and your baby will be safe even if they have a fever. In fact, pediatricians have been overdoing it. Until the past few decades, it was standard practice that any infant under three months old with a temperature above 38°C (100.4°F) or below 36.5°C (97.7°F) needed a full set of tests—including a spinal tap—and a few days of antibiotics until lab tests came back showing that they didn't have a bacterial infection. However, starting in the 1980s, research has confirmed what pediatricians already suspected: We worry way more about babies than we need to. Changes to practice have been piecemeal, with some centers altering their approach earlier than others as the data continued to emerge. By the late 1990s, pediatricians generally saved their worry for babies less than two months old, beginning to make decisions for babies one to two months old based on more individualized risk assessments.

The studies are ongoing, and our approach continues to evolve. But there's already awesome new science that's helping pediatricians decide how we can accurately identify which fevering babies do need poking and prodding. Hospital pediatricians around the country (me!) now use data from a national study to help us better predict which babies with fevers have viruses and which have bacterial infections. A key risk factor is age, so the modern baby who is one month old or younger will still likely get a complete workup. But for infants older than one month, we use a combination of other risk factors to decide which fevering babies need a complete workup and a hospital stay. Babies who don't have risk factors like prematurity, previous NICU stays, or abnormal lab tests rarely need a full set of tests and a hospital stay or just-in-case antibiotics.

Too much data? Don't stress, I got you covered. Here's how I've translated all that sexy science into the recommendations I give to friends and family when they ask about having visitors over during those first few months.

- **The first month is the riskiest, so it makes sense to limit visitors during this time period (even if covid exposure risk is low where and**

when you read this)—I said *limit*, not ban. Even in a post-pandemic world, there will be a need to keep tabs on which visitors are allowed over. Everyone is different in how much they crave company, and I'm not pressuring any introverts to open their doors before they are ready. But for parents like me, whose postpartum worries only subsided with the comfort and support of my friends and family, safely maximizing visitation is key. Just view it as a VIP list, and only grant your innermost circle entry through the velvet ropes to your newborn's nursery.

• **It's okay to have some restrictions (and require proof of immunization from anyone who wants to cuddle your baby)**—Barring a positive nasal swab, if you, another parent, or any primary caretaker has a cold, try not to stress: The importance of skin-to-skin contact, the immune benefits of breastfeeding (if that's what you're doing), and early bonding all outweigh the risks of your baby catching your germs. I've had to free many well-meaning parents from their self-inflicted "quarantine" to the guest room for a common cold and place their much-missed baby back into their arms. Wearing a mask, washing your hands, avoiding face kisses while you're actively sick are also all great strategies that can help minimize the chances you pass your sniffles on to your newborn. There are more serious viruses, however—like measles, pertussis, flu, and of course SARS-CoV-2—that *do* justify some distance. With the exception of a breastfeeding parent, it makes a lot of sense for a flu or covid-stricken caretaker to minimize snuggles when able and be extra diligent with their own mask-wearing.

If someone who isn't a primary caretaker or crucial member of the home support system (like a visiting grandparent, nanny, or someone critical to maintaining your postpartum sanity) has another type of cold virus, even if they text you a screenshot of their negative covid PCR test, it's still fine to delay their visit. In the first month, there's no need to risk your baby getting a fever from some sniffling houseguest out of politeness. Emily Post will understand.

Vaccines are also a must. Not just for your baby, but for everyone who comes in contact with them. This means requiring that all visitors are fully up-to-date not only on all routine vaccines (which might mean an MMR booster if they were born before 1967, when the vaccine schedule was different), but have also received the seasonal flu shot, the whooping cough booster, and yes, their covid vaccine. This was nonnegotiable for me, and it's also what my physician colleagues universally expect. One new mother and fellow pediatrician detailed how she had found the perfect nanny for her newborn, only to find out days before starting that she refused to get the flu shot. That was the only deal-breaker she had ever encountered, and a frantic search for replacement childcare was a no-brainer.

I encourage every family I counsel to make the same demand. A newborn can't start their set of childhood vaccines—the ones that protect against pneumonia, meningitis, and which have dropped infant mortality rates to the low levels they are today—until they are two months old, and the first round isn't even complete until six months of age. This final series includes whooping cough—a disease merely inconvenient to older children and adults, but often fatal to newborns. Babies also can't get their flu vaccine until they are six months old, and while influenza is miserable for everyone, the most common group that actually dies from it is infants. We'll take a much deeper dive into how crucial it is to protect babies against these vaccine-preventable diseases—which now includes covid!—in Chapter 9. For now, feel free to enforce the "no-vaccines, no-visit" policy with all your family and friends.

I remember counseling one mother—whose one-month-old daughter Maria was hospitalized for a bad cold—on how she could prevent her baby from getting so sick again. I explained that viruses are everywhere and unavoidable. But by requiring everyone who held her daughter to be fully immunized, she'd be able to protect her from some of the most serious infections out there. I completely understood her reluctance to engage her in-laws, friends, and family in a discussion of their own health. But I reminded her that it wasn't just their own health anymore: It was also Maria's. To put it bluntly, anyone who wasn't willing to get a few quick vaccines at their local pharmacy to protect her newborn's life probably hadn't earned the privilege of snuggling her. She made her round of phone calls before hospital discharge, assuring that every loving grandparent, aunt, uncle, and cousin could give as many cuddles as they wanted without sacrificing Maria's safety.

- **Just be a little cleaner than usual**—Placing a Costco-sized bottle of hand sanitizer on every surface of my house (not my most subtle hint) may have been overkill. But people are gross. You'd be surprised how even after years of covid-inspired hand-hygiene PSAs, plenty of people still don't realize that the fingers they placed on that subway rail are now covered in the best germs the city has to offer.

  This doesn't mean you need to disinfect your home top to bottom every time a guest arrives. It's just that sometimes people need a gentle reminder about some of the basics of infectious disease prevention. Handwashing is huge, and easy to make a part of your baby-holding routine. Have visitors wash their hands when coming into your home, and place a bottle of hand sanitizer next to your cuddle couch to be used before individual snuggle sessions. Yes, I've stopped friends from picking up my baby until they Purelled. No, it did not ruin our friendship.

Masks are also a great tool. During the 2020 covid surges, pediatricians saw an enormous drop in infant infections, notably flu and RSV. These viruses are two of the biggest culprits in giving newborns those fevers and serious breathing problems that earn them a trip to the hospital, so watching these bad bugs take a break was a true pandemic silver lining. We also saw over the next year how effective masks were (or weren't, if people didn't wear them) at keeping these infections at bay. All to say, witnessing the real-world effects of mask-wearing around newborns has been eye-opening. It's not black-or-white, and I don't think you need a blanket "no mask, no entry" rule for anyone coming to see your new bundle of joy. But I do think it's another helpful tool, especially during RSV and flu season. Whether it's asking visitors to keep their masks on when indoors, put them on only for close snuggles, or have a box of masks next to your cuddle couch, you should feel free to enforce whatever face-covering protocols feel safest in your home. You set the limits that make sense for your family, and you can always let your visitors know that their masks can come off for photo-ops—and that their social media feeds will be none the wiser.

Is It Safe? When (and How, and How Much) You Can Bring Your Baby Out and About

The first risk of taking a baby to explore the brave new world is the same as having visitors, since the great outdoors are full of people who are full of germs. RSV, influenza, and COVID-19—the possible exposures are seemingly endless. And it is much harder to control these exposures beyond the comfort of your own home. It's why I prioritized asking people over rather than venturing out for the first month. I also forced myself to hand my daughter off to my husband, mother, or other caretaker for a few hours and leave the house every few days, even just to grab lunch on my own or meet a friend downtown.

Having people over only gets you so far, and sometimes solo trips are great but not always feasible. If you're craving more time with your baby, or simply don't have the backup childcare to escape, it makes sense to favor locations where infectious exposure can be minimized. Friends' houses are great, and I was not shy about bringing over a Pack 'n Play and making myself at home for an afternoon to experience precious (fully vaccinated) adult conversation while my baby napped.

I was also more cautious when venturing out to crowded areas, especially during cold and flu season (the year was 2017, influenza was my greatest fear, and COVID-19 was but a distant, unknown nightmare). I still went for walks to the grocery store when it was warm enough, limiting her exposure to others by wearing her in the baby carrier instead of pushing her in a stroller. This is great for temperature regulation (we'll talk about that below), and also helps keep people from physically fawning over your little one. It's amazing how much others respect adult personal space over that of infants.

Higher-risk categories are ultra-crowded places (shopping malls during the holidays or library story hour were not our scene for the first month) and places where the risk of specific infections are more likely—like anywhere there's a known flu, measles, and, of course, covid outbreak.

Air travel is a special subcategory, and because my daughter was born during a flu epidemic, with multiple infant mortalities, I delayed my plane trip to visit extended family until flu season was over, when my baby was five months old. But others will need to fly earlier, and so I counsel families to consider plane travel on a case-by-case basis. In general, waiting until after two months makes a lot of sense to me because that's when your baby will have their first round of vaccines and be out of the clear not only for needing a spinal tap, but also for pretty much any other major testing if they get a fever.

The second risk to venturing outdoors is braving the elements. Exposure to hot and cold weather adds a whole new layer of worry. Exactly how dangerous this is remains unclear. We know that tiny babies aren't great at regulating their own body temperature—their big heads, low body-fat content, large area of exposed skin compared to their body size, and developing brains all make maintaining body heat more challenging than it is for you or me. This is why babies go under warming lights, get towel dried, and then have their temperatures checked every few hours after they are born. But there's little concrete data showing when, for how long, and at what temperatures babies can go outside without getting too hot or too cold. There is, however, a ridiculous, hilarious, and enraging collection of blog posts on the topic. One of my patients, after googling whether it was okay to bring her baby out for a walk on a warm summer day, found a site that confidently assured her she was free to take her baby out—as long as the temperature was exactly 80°F or lower. She spent weeks stuck inside, feeling unsafe to even meet friends at the local coffee shop, until she and I were able to reason why this arbitrary cutoff, based on zero evidence, made zero sense. After three weeks of isolation, armed with a plan to appropriately check for overheating and two clip-on fans attached to her baby's stroller, she was finally able to feel comfortable ignoring the baseless online fearmongering and join her friends for Sunday brunch a mere two blocks away.

Having a winter baby during one of the iciest seasons on record in Michigan meant my weather worries were of the opposite variety. For the first two weeks, I kept my daughter inside except for doctors' visits. I had to carefully balance my (in)sanity with my desire to not risk any further loss of body heat in my tiny, seemingly so fragile, newborn. Here's how I made my decision, and what I decided:

1. If a baby is warm or cold because of temperature exposure, they should be able to get back to normal when they go inside and get some quality skin-to-skin contact. I therefore tried to do as much

baby wearing as possible when I went out, because holding babies tight is the best way to keep their temperature controlled.

2. In babies under a month old, we can't tell if their temperature is the result of an infection without performing invasive testing, so I exercised more caution until my baby's one-month birthday. But after that, barring the occasional polar vortex, I felt comfortable taking her out and about more or less as much as I pleased.

3. In that first month, there will still be instances where the benefits of going out into the heat or cold will be worth it. A two-block walk with a newborn in 88°F weather may come with a small risk of overheating, but the ability to engage in normal activity and precious adult conversation is often worth it.

It's important to remember that pediatricians are making these risks vs. benefits assessments all the time, even in ways they might not realize. When I had to take my daughter in for a weight check and jaundice measurement on the fourth day of her life, that meant dressing her warmly, strapping her into her car seat, and braving the -15°F record cold that day for the run from the parking lot to the doctor's office, exposing her to sick kids at the pediatrician's office, and then doing the whole thing all over again for the trip home. This was a lot of exposure, and more than I ended up giving her for nonmedical outings for many weeks. If pediatricians understand that there are instances where it makes sense to risk braving the great outdoors, it's unfair (and untrue) to say the only worthwhile reason for this exposure is to come to our offices. It's why my framework lets you make the same risk-and-benefit assessment that pediatricians make when they decide when babies really do need to brave the elements. You should feel empowered to make those same decisions, embracing the many good reasons that will bring you out of your home.

Times have changed. We no longer have "villages" to raise our children, and modern parents are increasingly isolated in the newborn period, often without the network of extended family and community that makes a longer nesting period both feasible and enjoyable. Parents frequently stagger parental leave, or have uneven parental leaves, and it's not uncommon for one parent to be the sole at-home caretaker starting as early as the second week of a baby's life. Imposing a universal parent and newborn non-covid quarantine is unfair and unhealthy. Worse than a fever, overheating, cold exposure, a spinal tap, antibiotics, or even just a bad cold virus is an isolated parent, physically and emotionally exhausted, who feels like they just might lose it. Your sanity matters, and it also helps your baby. A parent's stress can impact not only how they are able to care for their little ones, but the behaviors and even the health of their infants. It's okay to embrace your own emotional well-being as just as important—perhaps even more important—as anything else.

THE BOTTOM LINE

5 out of 5 Pediatrician Parents Agree

- There are no official rules about when it's okay to host visitors and leave the house—we have to make some assumptions and do our best to balance the risks (exposure to heat, cold, and germs) with the benefits (people need to socialize!).

- The first month is the riskiest—it's when babies are most likely to need hospital stays if they have a fever, get sicker from viruses, and get too hot or cold if they go outside.

- It makes sense to limit visitors and travel in the first month, even in a world where #stayathome is no longer the official rule. Stick to a VIP list of people who can come over. It's okay to ban sick visitors unless they are primary caretakers.

- Everyone who comes near your baby needs their full set of vaccines, including the seasonal flu shot, covid shot, and all boosters (especially making sure that Tdap, MMR, pneumococcus, and shingles are up-to-date).

- Outdoor trips in the first month are okay, but be mindful of the weather (there are no hard rules on what temperatures are allowed, just try to hold your baby to your body as much as possible and use common sense). Avoid super-crowded areas, especially during cold and flu season, even when covid dangers fade into the background.

- Just be a little cleaner than usual. Anyone holding your newborn needs to wash their hands before snuggles, pandemic or none. Masks are also a great tool to help visitors protect your little one from all sorts of cough and cold viruses, especially in the first month.

4

FIFTY SHADES

....

How to Decipher the Rainbow Colors
of Baby Poop

One of the strangest rites of passage in becoming a parent is learning to spend a good portion of your day talking about poop. And you'd be surprised just how much there is to discuss. A week rarely goes by that I don't receive a text with a photo of a friend's beautiful new baby's dirty diaper, captioned with the famous three words: "Is this normal?"

It makes sense. If I hadn't been a pediatrician, my daughter's first bowel movements would have completely freaked me out. My non-physician husband's brows furrowed consistently during those first diaper changes, and I realized just how much I took for granted with my built-in baby knowledge. It's time to demystify infant poop *before* it shows up on your changing table (and clothes, and couch, and plenty of other places, sorry). Let's go through the colors (and shapes, and sizes, and frequency) of the baby poop rainbow you never thought you'd need to know, and which warning signs might indicate issues requiring medical care.

A common cause of (usually unnecessary) diaper concern is color. As a quick primer, baby's first poops are black and sticky. As your baby drinks milk and starts digesting it, their stool turns yellow and seedy. Over the next weeks to months, they become less seedy and turn some fun colors. Green, light brown, dark brown, yellow-brown, yellow-green, green-gray, yellow-gray—anything in this color palette is normal. There are basically only three colors that could be a source of concern (but often still aren't) and require some expert interpretation.

The first is intuitive. Red is the color of blood. When a baby's poop looks bright red, or has streaks of bright red, that's probably blood. This sounds scary, but streaks of blood can mean that a baby is simply constipated (causing skin to break down as they strain to pass stool, something that happens almost exclusively with older infants) or suffering from a bad diaper rash. It can also mean that a baby's gut isn't able to break down the protein in cow's milk (known as "milk protein intolerance"). If you see a small amount of red in your happy baby's diaper, and your baby isn't constipated or the streaks don't go away, it's a good idea to keep track of what a breastfeeding parent and baby are eating, make an appointment with the pediatrician, and come up with a plan from there. Large amounts of blood mean there could be active bleeding in a baby's belly, and your instinct to head to the emergency room is spot on.

The next "red flag" is actually a black one. I remember when my daughter was about ten months old and I asked the nanny how her day went. She told me they had had a wonderful time, but her diaper did look odd. Does she ever have poops that are black? My pediatrician brain jumped into overdrive and my heart raced: Did my baby have melena? Melena, you see, is the medical word for stool that has digested blood in it. It looks pitch-black, with a coarse, gravelly consistency. I responded instinctively as if I were on the hospital floors taking care of a patient. Did she save the diaper? Could I look at it?

As I reined back my interrogation, I remembered to take a look at the patient—I mean, my daughter. She was happy, smiling, playing with blocks. I said goodbye to my nanny, then sat on the floor for some quality baby time. A few hours later, she had another dirty diaper. When I opened it, it did indeed look black. I held it to the sunlight for my forensic inspection. I saw a dark blue tinge and some tiny peels. I laughed. My daughter had clearly eaten blueberries for breakfast. When you spend so much time interpreting every one of a baby's bodily functions, it can be hard to remember that most changes are normal. Digested blueberries look black. Beets look bright red. A whole slew of fun foods look orange, green, yellow, and gray.

Light gray stools—as in almost white—are the third color that merit a doctor's visit because they could signify rare liver problems. Otherwise, chances are that the rainbow coming out below is just a reflection of the colors that are going in above.

As a professional pediatrician and worry-prone mother, I too have spent a fair amount of time overthinking my baby's bowel movements. But dirty diapers aren't tea leaves, and there's usually no big message hidden inside them. It's okay not to agonize over your infant's poop palette. And if at the end of the day you're still worried, or just want to chat with someone who is as excited to talk about what the tint and texture of your baby's bowel movements could mean, that's okay too! Remember, you can call your pediatrician at any point and make a visit dedicated exclusively to scrolling through a museum exhibit's worth of dirty diaper photos.

It's not just colors that are the source of angst; there are endless blogs, advertisements, and practitioners ready to convince you that your baby's totally normal poop schedule is abnormal. It's not. In our world of mounting parental anxiety, we pediatricians see an increasing number of perfectly healthy babies whose parents have been told their babies have worrisome stool patterns. Most commonly, the concern is constipation. But in reality, most of these babies are just fine.

In the first month, after those dirty diapers have turned seedy and yellow, babies usually poop a lot. A lot can be *a lot*—like with every single feed, or more, maybe even a dozen times each day! Some babies, on the other hand, don't poop quite as much at first and might even start out with one dirty diaper every day, or even every other day. After the first few weeks, frequency usually decreases, and there are plenty of healthy babies who have a dirty diaper only once each week.

Constipation in babies in the first months of life is extremely rare. Since frequency is so variable, and because almost all babies grunt, strain, and even turn red while they pass bowel movements (it's not their fault, they just physically do not know how to relax their bumholes!), the only real sign

73

that your baby *might* be constipated in the first six months of life is consistently seeing dry, hard, or pellet-like poops. If this happens (which is still unlikely but is something we do see from time to time, primarily with formula-fed babies), just call your pediatrician and set up a time to chat. There's likely nothing serious going on, but they'll help you decide if any workup or treatment is needed.

Once your baby starts solid foods, usually around six months, things will change again. Your baby will still get the majority of their nutrition and hydration from breast milk and/or formula, and up until about one year of age the foods they eat are mostly for sensory, motor, and taste exploration. However, some parents do find that the combination of some harder-to-digest solid foods and a decrease in the amount of breast milk/formula their baby consumes causes constipation. Again, the most common cases I see are completely healthy babies who simply have less frequent and more formed bowel movements, as is expected. But actual constipation does happen in this six-to-twelve-month age group. The good news is that it's still extremely overdiagnosed by understandably anxious parents who have been told to scrutinize their baby's diapers and worry constantly that something might be wrong.

And of course, the internet is eagerly waiting to push unnecessary and even dangerous interventions. I can't even begin to count how many parents try to help happy and healthy babies poop more often due to this faulty information. One family was so worried that weekly bowel movements meant their five-month-old baby was constipated that they went overboard with giving her water to drink. And while water does help soften bowel movements, it also can cause dangerously low levels of salts (like sodium) in the blood, especially in little babies. This poor family ended up with a trip to the hospital for IV sodium, where I met them and explained that their happy, growing baby was pooping as much as she needed to.

In the end, it's important to remember that your infant is probably not constipated. Try not to focus on the frequency of dirty diapers or how much your poor little poop-maker grunts and moans, or how their cheeks turn red and purple during bathroom breaks. Shut out the noise and remember just one thing: If your baby starts to have hard, or pellet-like, dry poops, call your pediatrician. You'll talk it out and avoid unnecessary laxatives, suppositories, prune juice, and anxiety-provoking Google searches.

In an effort to make parenting officially impossible, the internet has also decided that new parents should worry about the exact opposite of constipation during needless diaper scrutiny: diarrhea. Just like with constipation, don't get worried about frequency—if your baby poops after every feed, you'll be in a normal if exhausting pattern of near-constant diaper changes. It's consistency that clues in pediatricians on whether or not there's cause for concern. After the first few weeks of seedy yellow poops, your baby's diaper will turn into a pudding-like mush. It's a gross but memorable description that pediatricians love to share with parents. Pasty poops are normal, and even loose stools are common in infants, especially in those first few weeks. If your baby's bowel movements are truly watery, that could be diarrhea. It's probably a cold virus, so your pediatrician will help you focus on making sure your baby stays hydrated while they recover with some extra snuggles. And if you're worried your baby is getting dehydrated, or just aren't sure, bring them into the doctor's office or emergency room! It's never your job to decide if your baby needs urgent medical care. Your worry is enough, and pediatricians are always here to take over.

In very, very rare cases, stool can be truly greasy or constantly watery, even when your baby isn't sick. This is another case where your pediatrician will work closely with you to see if this is just how your baby's intestines work, or if there's an actual problem with absorbing food and fluids. There are almost always other signs. Babies who don't get enough nutrition have problems gaining weight, and babies who can't get enough liquid from milk or formula become dehydrated. Again, it's not your job to sort through it. True problems are uncommon, and your pediatrician will take the reins and decide if there's any testing that should be done.

Baby bowel movements are a surprising source of parental anxiety, but they don't have to be. Yes, you can always call your baby's doctor with any concern, and if something just doesn't seem right or you just aren't sure, please reach out! But it's also important to remember there is no need to feel panicked at each diaper change. There are so many shapes, colors, sizes, and frequencies of dirty diapers that are truly normal. When you're done wiping your baby's adorable bottom, don't obsess, don't stress, and just throw that dirty diaper in the garbage where it belongs.

THE BOTTOM LINE

5 out of 5 Pediatrician Parents Agree

- Baby poop comes in all shapes, sizes, and colors, but the (possibly) worrisome colors are red, black, and white.

- Babies don't need to poop every day—as long as baby poops are soft and don't seem to be painful, your baby is very unlikely to be constipated.

- All babies strain when they poop; this also doesn't mean they're constipated.

- Diarrhea is also overdiagnosed. Some babies poop a dozen times a day. True watery or greasy stools are something to talk about with your pediatrician. This could indicate something as simple as a cold virus, so chat with your baby's doctor early and don't get caught up in unnecessary worry.

- Try not to obsess too much over diapers; remember that what comes out below is just a reflection of what goes in above!

5

A PAIN IN THE BEHIND

• •

How to Prevent and Treat
Diaper Rash and Keep Your
Baby's Sensitive Skin Happy

When I came home from the hospital with my sweet and exhausting bundle of joy, the last thing on my mind was skin care. Having recited the "newborn discharge talk" more times than I could count during my rotations in the newborn nursery, I knew that bathing could wait. Newborns shouldn't get submerged baths until their umbilical cords fall off, and after that it's not that important. As I've told countless parents, babies are pretty clean. Bathing a few times a week, maybe even less, is more than enough.

But even though it shouldn't have, my daughter's diaper rash caught me by surprise. What started as a little bit of red quickly evolved into raw, bleeding skin. Being born early means that body parts aren't fully developed, and skin is no exception. All babies are born a little undercooked (a product of our evolutionary history and the reason human newborns are even more fragile than those of many other species), so it is truly the rare baby who doesn't have some diaper irritation. Also, diapers hold urine and stool, which is not meant to sit on human skin. Even the most vigilant, obsessive parent can't change every single diaper the moment a baby fills it. The result: Almost every single baby will have a diaper rash at some point.

Whether it's everyday redness, a serious rash, dry skin, or eczema, it turns out that newborn skin can be pretty high-maintenance. Never fear, I'm here to share all the pediatrician trade secrets to maintaining the healthiest skin. It's one of the most common topics encountered by pediatricians, and a surprising challenge for a huge number of new parents.

What's the Best Way to Prevent and Treat Those Pesky Diaper Rashes that Just Won't Seem to Go Away?

Let's start with baby bum care, a fairly straightforward topic that I've seen cause unnecessary worry. The glut of information available certainly hasn't helped. The booming baby product market has more options for diapers, wipes, creams, soaps, and lotions than ever before. Parenting blogs indulge obsessions: How red is your baby's bottom? Are you using the right diaper cream? That bum brush to spread Desitin like cake frosting is an absolute must. Buy only brand-name products, shop organic, spend more time, spend more money, look at your baby's butt all day and every day.

In my office I saw a father who had purchased one of every type of ointment on the market. Examining his beautiful new baby, I saw a diaper filled with clear goop, pasty white, and poop mixed in. I asked him if his baby had a particularly bad rash he was trying to fix. No, but he heard this was how to prevent it. We wiped off the layers to see red, angry skin after days of this "preventive" routine. A third-year resident, I had rotated with pediatric dermatologists, expert general pediatricians, and now had extensive personal experience with my own baby's bleeding bottom. We cleaned my adorable patient up and started over.

While there are certainly good arguments for routine use of diaper cream, there are plenty who use barrier treatments more judiciously. In the end, it's all about how they're used. It's really the technique of cleaning, layering, and exposing skin to air that makes the most difference. Each baby is different, but most tiny bottoms do best with a regimen that minimizes irritation. For my daughter, this meant using a spray bottle of plain water to clean off stool, then dabbing with simple, unscented "water wipes" as a finishing touch. When I had time, I'd keep her diaper open and place her in front of a fan for as long as possible. Before closing that diaper back up, I would take a huge glop of zinc oxide and apply that thick, "frosting-like" layer as generously as my fingers or bum brush would allow. I ended the routine with a top coat of A&D or Vaseline (petroleum jelly), which I found helpful in keeping the diaper from sticking to her frosted white bottom. And when it was time for the next diaper change, I made sure to remove the next inevitable layer of poop as gingerly as I could, keeping as much of that double cream barrier intact as possible.

I would classify my own personal regimen as relatively intensive compared to many other perfectly acceptable routines. It was necessary for my daughter's fragile, premature, rash-prone skin. But it's entirely possible that your baby's bottom will do just fine with a thin layer of petroleum jelly, a quick dab of zinc oxide to redder areas, or nothing besides a few open-to-air sessions per day. There's always a little trial and error, and you'll quickly learn what your baby likes best. When troubleshooting, though, remember to check in with your pediatrician to see if there's any medical, treatable reason for your skin struggles. And also remember that limiting irritation (replace aggressive wiping with fragrance-free dabbing and spraying), maximizing aeration (why yes, those are Wee-Wee Pads intended for puppy toilet training that I've placed under my daughter's bare bottom, thank you for asking), and sticking to the basics (I repeat, zinc oxide and petroleum jelly/A&D are all you need) can fix almost all diaper-care issues.

The other secret? Setting realistic expectations. It's the exception, not the rule, to have a newborn whose bottom is completely rash-free. Without signs of infection and with a happy and growing baby, diaper irritation does not signal a terrible, uncaring parent. Despite my most valiant efforts, I was never able to get my newborn's bum completely free of redness or even areas of skin breakdown until biology kicked in and her epidermis toughened up. So if that pesky redness hangs around until your little one literally grows a thicker skin, that's okay.

When, How, and How Frequently Does My Baby Need a Bath?

The newborn "cheat sheet" that you'll leave the hospital with covers the first few weeks of basic care and hygiene and is reasonably uncontroversial. Until your baby's umbilical cord falls off, avoid submerged baths and simply wipe them down with a wet towel when you want to, and only if you want to. Newborn skin also looks dry, wrinkly, and even flaky for several weeks (remember that uterine hot tub they just came out of?), so don't be alarmed. Resist the temptation to use lotions, ointments, and other unnecessary moisturizers that are at best a waste of money and at worst can cause irritation.

That's nice and straightforward, but how should you keep your little one fresh and clean after their umbilical cord falls off? The short answer is that babies stay pretty clean, and bathtime should be as frequent an occurrence as you and your baby want it to be. The longer answer starts with a pediatric dermatology PowerPoint lecture on infant skin layers, moisture, and decades of bathing philosophy (no, really, I confirmed this with pediatric dermatologist friends), and then ends with the same conclusion. Unless your baby has an actual skin moisture problem like eczema (stay tuned!), you can bathe them as much or as little as makes sense to you. There are plenty of seasoned pediatric dermatologists who swear that daily bathing followed by head-to-toe emollient (like Vaseline or the generic petroleum jelly equivalent) keeps moisture locked in and is the best for all baby skin. Many others say that since bathing dries out skin (when water evaporates it takes the skin's moisture with it, making bathtime a counterintuitively dehydrating part of your skin care regimen), less is more. I fell into the second camp and bathed my daughter about once or twice a week for her first year of life. Are your eyes wide? Most parents are shocked when I confess this! I'm not offended; I know my daughter was perfectly clean and cared for. But with a baby market pushing bathtime gadgets, toys, gear, lotions, and potions for frequently bathed skin, it's easy to forget that infants, even those who cruise and groove around your home, are just not all that dirty.

The other main motivator for my less-is-more bathing regimen was that my daughter hated her baths. No gizmo or fancy tub helped, toys were thrown, parents were splashed, tears were shed by all. She simply screamed and cried every single time, and bathtime was not a fun family event or relaxing part of her bedtime routine. So we just started doing it less frequently, and everyone was happier.

What Does the Word "Eczema" Actually Mean, and Is It the Same as Dry Skin?

It's time to review the difference between eczema and normal baby dry skin—probably the most important distinction when deciding if, when, and what to put on your baby's scaly, itchy skin.

Parents and pediatricians alike commonly use the word "eczema" to refer to a certain type of skin condition that is technically called "atopic dermatitis." I've heard run-of-the-mill dry skin called "eczema," which is totally fine outside of pediatric dermatology clinical rotations. I'm not here to grade anyone on the precision of their medical terminology. Just know that because the cause is different, the treatment is as well. Regular old skin dryness, even if severe, just needs more moisture. Atopic dermatitis needs this too, but we pediatricians have some more tricks up our sleeve to help as well.

Pediatricians sit through countless lectures on the causes

of and treatments for atopic dermatitis, and pediatric dermatologists sit through countless more. While we don't know exactly what causes it, we do know that it occurs when skin cells become inflamed from some convergence of immune dysregulation, skin barrier dysfunction, and skin irritation.

How will you know if your baby has super-dry skin or actual atopic dermatitis? Your pediatrician will tell you, of course! Both are helped by increasing skin moisture, so if you suspect your little one's skin lies somewhere on the everyday dry to angry atopic dermatitis spectrum, there are some easy changes that will help no matter where the diagnosis lands. These will also be the first changes your pediatrician and/or pediatric dermatologist recommend, so now you can show up to your appointments having already done the first homework assignment (it's okay, being a nerd is so hot these days!). Feel free to:

1. Frequently and liberally apply 100% petroleum jelly (warning! "Vaseline baby" and other deceptively marketed products often have fragrance)

2. Avoid fragranced diapers, wipes, soaps, lotions, creams, and anything that touches your baby's skin

3. Limit the duration of baths, keeping them warm rather than hot, and slather that petroleum jelly all over lightly toweled, damp skin right away, before the water has a chance to evaporate.

This will likely help, maybe even a whole lot. Even so, you'll want to keep that pediatrician appointment to fully debrief, discuss, diagnose, and move forward. There's no need to go down a rabbit hole of atopic dermatitis treatment that's unnecessary, or travel down one alone if that's the true diagnosis.

If My Breastfeeding Baby Has Eczema, Do I Really Have to Cut Foods Out of My Diet?

Nope. This is an easy one to answer, and a source of needless maternal sacrifice. Babies with dry or sensitive skin *don't* get better when parents change formulas or make their own diets more restricted, and anyone telling you this is the way to go is simply wrong. And for babies with real atopic dermatitis, there's no need to eliminate foods unless there's a clear reason to do so. Atopic dermatitis is related to food allergies, so babies with this diagnosis *do* tend to have more actual allergies and real food reactions. If you notice a consistent pattern where certain foods are triggering reactions, talk to your pediatrician, pediatric dermatologist, and/or pediatric allergist. They'll help you decide if testing makes sense and if/when/how to eliminate certain foods from your diet.

If you're thinking, *What's the harm in testing, isn't more information better?*—I totally get that. So many tests, including skin-prick testing for allergies, are marketed directly to parents. Whether they're selling you an at-home rapid testing kit or pushing you to ask your pediatrician about testing, they're out to make money. There's a role for skin prick and blood tests to diagnose allergies, but not without a doctor's assessment and discussion. The biggest risk to "more information" is that it's confusing or wrong information. False positives and uncertain answers are very common, and there's no need to start taking away nutritious and delicious foods from you and your baby if they aren't a problem to begin with. What's more, we now know that early exposure to allergens is super important in *preventing* food allergies. Unnecessarily eliminating common food allergy triggers, especially in kids who are more likely to develop food allergies in the first place, ironically increases their risk of having serious allergic problems in the future.

Are Those Special Soaps and Lotions Worth Your Precious Time and Money?

If you've been on the internet today, my guess is you've already seen a targeted ad for a baby soap, wash, shampoo, lotion, or ointment. I'm sure you've also already received samples and coupons in the mail as part of a registry completion gift or other expecting-parent promotion.

Yet for most babies, lotion will stay optional even after their uterine-hot-tub wrinkles have disappeared. A minimalistic approach, starting with fewer products and adding in moisturizers as necessary, will save your pocketbook and sanity. Whether it's dry skin or severe atopic dermatitis, maximizing moisture and minimizing irritants are the name of the game. Of course, nothing simple is ever simple when it comes to baby product marketing, and parents now have to wade through a sea of "for eczema" products that are actually full of scents, irritants, and additives. Since babies with atopic dermatitis commonly have the type of allergic reactions that happen when an irritant touches the skin, literally anything can cause a reaction (even the lanolin in Aquaphor, or Vaseline that comes with a mild fragrance).

So while there are some brands of lotions and soaps that are better than others, it's not always the ones you think. A pediatric dermatologist I work with once saw a baby come in with the angriest, reddest skin she had seen in months. This six-month-old's parents had been diligent with their simple and "clean" regimen—twice weekly baths and daily head-to-toe "natural" moisturizer from a high-end grocery chain. They showed their doctor the bottle: only organic ingredients, all from plants such as *rhus toxicodendron*. With an encyclopedic knowledge of skin irritants, the dermatologist cracked the case immediately. Incredibly enough, this popular "healthy" market peddles topical treatments that are made with poison ivy. As extreme an example as this might seem, I've seen similar product confusion and unnecessary, even dangerous, skin care with my patients and among my friends.

Pediatric dermatologists have a consistent list of the brands that pass the simple-ingredient test, and it's a short list. For the majority of babies, the only items you'll want in their toiletry kit are an unscented cleanser (Dove is a dermatologist fan favorite) and—all together now—the least expensive, off-brand, Costco-sized tub of unscented 100% petroleum jelly you can get your hands on. Lotions are too watery to effectively moisturize and are always diluted with something irritating (often alcohol!), so you can just say no. When it's time to moisturize, there's rarely a need to use anything other than unscented petroleum jelly. A few other ointments and creams (certain Cetaphil, Vanicream, and CeraVe products) rank as distant runners-up if your Vaseline grease-down gets a little too, well, greasy. Some families swear by coconut oil, which seems to be okay too, as long as your baby isn't allergic. And like with diaper rashes, technique is everything. Whether it's everyday dryness or serious atopic dermatitis, the path to success is paved with unscented goop—that covers your baby head to toe, right after their bath, with as much moisture and love sealed in as is possible.

THE BOTTOM LINE

5 out of 5 Pediatrician Parents Agree

- Almost every baby has a diaper rash, so try not to stress too much over a little bit of redness and irritation.

- The best diaper rash treatment and prevention is a simple barrier cream, maximizing open-to-air time, and skipping fancy goops and medicated ointments unless your pediatrician prescribes them.

- Babies don't get very dirty; bathing weekly (or as often as is fun for the whole family) is plenty.

- From dry skin to medical eczema, prioritizing skin hydration is key. Focusing on locking in moisture after baths with petroleum jelly is the way to go. Avoiding fragrances and irritants is helpful too.

- If you're worried your baby has medical eczema (atopic dermatitis), check in with your pediatrician before diving down the rabbit hole of treatments. Elimination diets are out, and simple petroleum jelly goopy-goodness is in. And there are countless fancy "for eczema" products that cause way more harm than good.

6

CO-SLEEP NO MORE

• •

The Truth about Safe Sleep Guidelines

Almost every pediatrician counsels new parents on by-the-book safe sleep. And while the Safe to Sleep campaign, mandating that infants sleep on their backs in an empty crib, has led to an impressive reduction in SIDS since the early 1990s, the reality is that few parents—even the pediatricians among them!—are able to consistently follow these rules. In this chapter, we'll take a deep dive into the ongoing SIDS research and give you a full understanding of why pediatricians recommend the stern guidelines they do. But then, unlike almost every other pediatrician-approved guide, I'm going to embrace how deeply unrealistic perfect safe sleep practices actually are. My own approach has been to encourage parents to set themselves up for by-the-book safe sleep. But I also do the unthinkable (at least in this country) and outline how parents can make bed-sharing safer.

During my residency training, I became passionate about safe sleep and SIDS prevention. In short, safe sleep is a movement to prevent sudden infant death syndrome (SIDS), a disease every bit as horrible as it sounds. I read studies, joined initiatives, provided counseling, and did everything I could to hopefully save as many tiny lives as possible. As a childless doctor, preaching official American Academy of Pediatrics guidelines was easy and seemed uncontroversial. Infants should never sleep in the same bed as anyone else and instead should always be put down alone, swaddled, and on their backs in an empty crib. At every visit, I recited this advice to new parents, which was met with smiles and nods. I smiled back, thinking that each interaction would save this family from unspeakable tragedy, entirely unaware of the reality each exhausted parent faced at home.

In my defense, my evangelical support of official safe sleep is based on good data. In the mid-1980s, two landmark scientific findings converged: In 1985, a team of researchers led by Dr. D. P. Davies demonstrated with hard data that in Hong Kong, where babies were routinely put to sleep on their backs, the rates of SIDS was much lower. Around the same time, laboratory research found that when babies sleep on their backs, their sleep brain waves act differently, allowing them to wake up more easily if something disturbs them (like forgetting to breathe, which is common in sleeping newborns). The medical community was sold on the science and acted quickly.

Over the next decade, a wave of public health campaigns swept the international community, spreading to the United States by 1992 under the name Back to Sleep. The messaging was simple: put babies on their back to sleep, always, no exceptions. From 1992 to 2002, there was a 50% decline in the number of SIDS cases in the United States, and it was hard to view Back to Sleep as anything but a godsend. Over the years, additional evidence-based strategies—babies must sleep alone in their crib, no blankets or toys, swaddle and pacifier only, in the same room as parents—have been folded in, and Back to Sleep was rebranded Safe to Sleep to incorporate these changes.

So, if official safe sleep saves lives—which it does—why are we still even talking about it? The main reason is because most parents don't consistently follow these recommendations. A CDC survey from 2009 to 2015 found that 61% of U.S. parents reported bed-sharing (co-sleeping actually means sharing the same space—room or bed—with your baby, although the terms "bed-sharing" and "co-sleeping" are often used interchangeably) as a routine practice. And pediatricians, the majority of whom follow official American Academy of Pediatrics guidelines when counseling families, are just as guilty: Every single one of my pediatrician-mother peers has admitted to bed-sharing.

One new mom, a friend and colleague, confessed to me that while she did her best to adhere to by-the-book safe sleep with her first child, she made no such attempt for her second. "I slept! And it made breastfeeding so much easier. I put the mattress on the floor, sent my husband to the guest room, and barely even woke up as she nursed throughout the night." I remember almost crying at the thought of this sleep-promoting bliss, and when she added that she "couldn't have survived a second baby without doing this," I believed her.

I've heard countless other stories highlighting just how hard it is to practice official safe sleep, and how doing so can even have negative consequences. I've also lived through it. It's not *physically* hard to swaddle a newborn, stick a pacifier in their mouth, and place them on their back on a firm bassinet mattress next to your bed. But they will almost certainly hate it. I remember my daughter, strapped into her straitjacket-like Halo-brand sleep-swaddle, flopping her head and feet up and down like a fish on land. You wouldn't have an easy time sleeping like this, and neither do newborns. Studies show that safe sleeping newborns wake up far more often than those who share a bed with parents. That means shorter stretches of sleep for babies, and shorter stretches of sleep for their caretakers.

It's no wonder that so many parents simply give up on Safe to Sleep—even those who initially set out to follow pediatrician guidelines. Being an exhausted parent is exhausting, and living this sleepless nightmare finally helped me understand why parents make the tough choice to abandon strict, evidence-based recommendations. Where I had previously judged parents harshly for seemingly risking their newborns' lives, I now understand that there are cases where having a sleepless caretaker is more dangerous than modifying by-the-book practices—yes, even including the possibility of bed-sharing.

Like my case. Even before the onset of my postpartum anxiety—which caused me to constantly worry that something awful, like SIDS, would happen to my baby—I insisted on practicing Safe to Sleep to the letter of the law. But this absolutely came at a cost. For the first three months of my daughter's life, I slept no more than three hours at a time. When she cried at night, hungry, I got out of bed, picked her up, unswaddled her, removed her pacifier, placed her skin to skin on my breast, fed her if she could latch or gave her a bottle if she couldn't, then repeated the Safe to Sleep routine all over again and crawled into bed. The sleep deprivation hit me like a slap in the face. My mood became more volatile, my worries deepened, and even the edges of my reality began to blur. I remember many a three a.m. wake-up, rocking my adorable, screaming baby in my intentionally uncomfortable chair (chosen to keep me awake), fantasizing about bringing her into my bed for the final three hours until my alarm went off. But the risk of SIDS loomed large, and I refused to change my routine.

The infant sleep conversation has been a polarized debate of equally dangerous extremes: by-the-book safe sleep vs. ditching science altogether for attachment parenting, decidedly unsafe bed-sharing. The pediatric community's refusal to meet parents where they are has left a craterous opening for predatory pseudoscientific websites, which are now the primary places exhausted parents can even find a discussion of bed-sharing techniques. I've read countless blogs offering advice on how to share a bed in some magical way that assures your baby could never have SIDS. What a coincidence that risk-free bed-sharing includes purchasing promoted co-sleeping products! Some counseling is more insidious: Evangelical lactation organizations often imply that the risk of SIDS drops to zero if mothers follow their safe bed-sharing rules—which of course include maximized breastfeeding.

But despite questionable motivation and misinformed messaging, the concept of safer bed-sharing is valid—and crucial to discuss. It's not that traditional safe sleep isn't safest—it is! That is, it is in an ideal world, in an optimal setup, in a situation in which parents have the structural and personal support to make this setup feasible and sustainable. For the majority of modern parents, however, that just isn't the reality we have been gifted. Modifying guidelines to meet individual family needs, and understanding that there will always be obstacles that make strict, by-the-book, adherence to safety measures impossible, isn't just kind—it's also evidence-based medicine. We call it "harm reduction," and we have tons of compelling research showing just how well it works (like how comprehensive sexual education is much better at preventing pregnancy and STI transmission than abstinence-only education, or how helping patients decrease tobacco intake leads to much better long-term health outcomes than pushing them to "just quit" at every visit).

Let's learn from all these great examples and ditch Safe to Sleep "bed-sharing abstinence only" education. Instead, you can count on embracing a more nuanced approach, still striving for by-the-book, safest safe sleep practices when you can, while having strategies to mitigate risk as much as possible when you can't. Here's the pediatrician-and-mom approved approach that I use when discussing safe sleep with my own patients. It's a framework you can actually follow, and one you can use to create a customized plan with your pediatrician that works for your individual situation. It's time to make sleep safer for the real babies of the world, not the theoretical ones in instructional handouts.

The Road Map for the Safest Sleep Possible (for an Actual Human Baby)

Safe "Safe Sleep" Is Still Safest

Embracing the nuances of bed-sharing doesn't mean ignoring decades of data, and there's no reason to pretend that Safe to Sleep doesn't exist. I still believe that in an ideal setup—where some confluence of adequate parental leave, social support, and serendipity prevent solo-sleeping from causing danger-ous parental exhaustion—Safe to Sleep is absolutely the best way to put a baby to bed. Even if bed-sharing is a likely or inevitable possibility, attempting safe sleep in earnest is worth-while. Before you bring your little one home, you should have an AAP-approved setup at the ready. An empty bassinet, crib, or Pack 'n Play, and some swaddle blankets or sleep-sacks are all you need to be fully prepared to give by-the-book, Safe to Sleep safe sleep an honest try.

Safe "Unsafe" Sleep Is Better than Unsafe "Safe" Sleep

Safe to Sleep has become so ingrained that the idea of break-ing it intentionally is much more terrifying than the reality of breaking it accidentally. But science strongly suggests the opposite. I know from countless discussions with friends, patient families, and of course from myself, that many of these strict Safe to Sleep abiding parents refuse to consider bed-sharing even after admitting to falling asleep on the couch. Data and clinical experience, however, shows that it is riskier to fall asleep even occasionally in a definitively unsafe setup (like sofas and chairs) than to more frequently sleep in an optimized bed-sharing arrangement. And the reality is that every parent, no matter how dedicated they may be (like me!) to strict Safe to Sleep practices, will have at least one (and likely many, many more) instances of slipping.

The other main harm of refusing to modify rigid Safe to Sleep practices is your own sleep deprivation in and of itself. Even if you don't fall asleep holding your baby on a decidedly less safe surface, it's an inescapable truth that a strict Safe to Sleep parent, especially one with a limited "village" of caretakers able to tag in for infant care, will be more exhausted than their bed-sharing counterpart. Parental exhaustion isn't "just" miserable. I know from my own experience just how much my physical and mental health suffered, and how much that impacted my ability to nurture and enjoy my newborn. Parental health *is* infant health, and we have to factor in measures that promote your own well-being into the risk vs. benefit assessment.

It also turns out that parental sleep deprivation is probably directly dangerous for babies as well. Newer research suggests that parental exhaustion might be a risk factor for SIDS itself. In a notable study that compared the sleeping habits of infants who died of SIDS to their healthy counterparts, having a parent who gets less than four hours of sleep in a row increased the chances of SIDS more than bed-sharing did. Though there is limited data available, it's a correlation worthy of important consideration, and something that aligns with what we see in the lab and in the real world. We know that how infants and parents synchronize their sleep-wake cycles is a key part of the biology of SIDS prevention, so any-thing that decreases parental responsiveness during sleep (including extreme exhaustion) would at least theoretically increase SIDS risk.

It's clear that most parents will benefit from having a bed-sharing setup ready when the risks from exhaustion become too great. So what does this setup look like? Fortu-nately, there is some science that can guide us in mitigating bed-sharing risk—even if there are only a handful of studies and the data is limited. These studies have shown that the link between bed-sharing and SIDS decreases dramatically if you remove other, larger risk factors, like having a parent who smokes or drinks alcohol, or using a duvet or comforter in bed. If you remove a few more risks—including overcrowded homes, those exhausted parents who sleep less than four hours, and being born premature—the correlation between bed-sharing and SIDS disappears in some studies altogether.

While this data isn't enough to change our official public health recommendations (yet), it's helped individual pediatri-cians and larger research groups to reevaluate how we counsel families about safe sleep. And there's evidence that replac-ing rigid, Safe to Sleep evangelism with customized "harm reduction" guidance has real benefits. In New Zealand, public health research and campaigns push pediatricians to focus on helping parents understand their personal risk fac-tors for SIDS. The next step—removing whatever risk factors they can—always includes a discussion of safer bed-sharing, assuming that it's something parents are considering or even already practicing. In the United Kingdom, there's been a similar nuance-embracing campaign. The results are impressive. New Zealand has seen a 30% decrease in SIDS deaths since 2010. In the United Kingdom, SIDS rates are down 40% since 2003. These are enviable statistics, as SIDS deaths in the United States have essentially plateaued after the post–Back to Sleep decline from 1992–2002.

You can absolutely do your very best to adhere to AAP-sanctioned solo-sleeping practices while still preparing for plan B. And the best time to prepare for something is *before* you need it. Here are the basics of how to make your own sleep space safer for your infant—just in case—so you never have to wake in a panic from accidental co-sleeping in a chair, couch, or other decidedly unsafe surface.

Mattresses need to be firm and low to the floor.

If you have a typical American bed, it's too high off the ground and almost certainly too soft. A lot of the arguments in favor of bed-sharing come from the fact that solo-sleeping is relatively new. Prior to the past few centuries, babies typically slept with their mothers, surrounded by a cocoon of SIDS-preventing carbon dioxide from mom's exhaled breaths, and breastfed throughout the night for further SIDS protection. So if we're going to use evolution to justify safer bed-sharing, we need to be honest with how parents and babies have slept over the course of history—which is on the floor and with minimal padding.

No blankets—really.

Studies on bed-sharing risk confirm what all pediatricians know from real-life tragedies: Thick blankets, duvets, comforters, and the like are all bad news. Invest in some footed pajamas for yourself (the zip-up ones are great for overnight breastfeeding!) and just use a thin blanket or sheet anytime you share a sleep space with your infant. Pillows should be small and come nowhere near your tiny baby's face. If you're reading this and think, "There's no way I'll be able to fall asleep on a firm mattress with just a sheet!" then bless you, you've never had a newborn.

Don't waste money on in-bed sleepers.

DockATots, in-bed sleepers, and other crazy bed-sharing contraptions are untested and unproven. The soft padding should be enough to give parents pause, but the marketing is compelling and insidious. While manufacturer labels warn that unsupervised sleep in these cushioned concave pillows can lead to suffocation death, this fine print is microscopic compared to the advertising. Instagram and Facebook posts almost always show them cradling a sleeping infant, leading parents—including mommy bloggers, who recommend them as a baby-bed in the same posts as actually safe-for-sleep bedside bassinets—to assume they make bed-sharing safer. The reality is that there are currently no bed-sharing devices that have even been tested by the Consumer Product Safety Commission, something websites like consumerreports.org (which we talked about in Chapter 2) rely on to decide if a product is safe for its intended use. In fact, we have data to suggest the opposite: In 2019, twelve cases of SIDS were tragically linked to "safer" bed-sharing devices. The only surface your infant should be on is a firm bassinet or crib mattress, or directly on your own firm mattress next to you.

But what about rolling over onto baby? Any way to prevent that?

Until we have safe in-bed sleepers, we have to rely on other strategies to protect babies. Having a mattress on the ground is great because babies can't roll off onto the floor, meaning you can more safely place them on the outside of the mattress and not between two people or between a person and the wall (both provide opportunities for baby to get wedged between things). If one parent is a biological mother, it's safest to place baby next to her. Mothers' bodies sync better with our infants, and we moms don't need any studies to tell us that we awaken much more easily and quickly, especially in those first few weeks.

No smokers, not now, not ever.

Secondhand smoke is one of the strongest risk factors for SIDS. This means that you should do everything you can to remove smoke exposure from your little one's life (yes, it's okay to ban Uncle Joe from visiting until he can at least go a few days without inhaling). It also means that babies who had smoke exposure in-utero, or who can't have smoke removed from their newborn lives altogether, are in a different risk category for SIDS, so striving for the safest sleep setup possible becomes even more important.

Bed-sharing isn't for party nights.

A big part of reducing the risks from bed-sharing means having parents, just like infants, remain in as much of a normal sleep pattern as possible. Studies show that alcohol consumption is a risk factor for SIDS, which makes a whole lot of sense. When alcohol and other sedatives are in your system, you can't connect your sleep-cycle with your baby in that magical way that reminds your baby to breathe. In addition, anything that dulls your awareness and reaction time makes it more likely that you'll roll over or otherwise unintentionally hurt your little one. The bottom line is that parents who share a sleep space with their infant should absolutely abstain from any sleep-disrupting substances, recreational or prescribed.

Back to Sleep is still king.

Placing infants on their backs still saves lives, even for babies who are on the same sleep surface as their parents. There's no evidence at all to support propping little heads up to prevent reflux, and similarly there's no need to put babies on their side to keep their heads round (some head flatness is inevitable and tummy time will prevent it from being a problem). Back to Sleep has consistently been shown to be critical in preventing SIDS, no matter where your baby sleeps. You absolutely do need to always put your baby on their back—next to you, not lying on your chest—every time, no matter what.

Safe Sleep Is a Moving Target

There will be times when strict Safe to Sleep is possible and even optimal. I count the first two weeks of my daughter's life as falling into this category. With my husband on paternity leave and my parents staying with us, there were enough able-bodied caretakers to practice Safe to Sleep without introducing dangerous levels of sleep-deprivation. But when it was just me, my completely overwhelmed state led to new risks. Looking back, I desperately wish that I had been given permission to embrace safer bed-sharing during the darkest times, when my depression and exhaustion introduced more risks than (more safely) sharing a sleeping space.

It's also crucial to look at all the risk factors together. Many parents—and even pediatricians—don't realize that these risk factors aren't the kind that add together; they multiply. This means that any baby who has more than one SIDS risk factor that can't be removed isn't a good candidate for bed-sharing at all. Yes, those parents should still understand that safer bed-sharing is better than falling asleep on a fluffy mattress or sofa. But in those cases, working harder toward exclusive Safe to Sleep becomes even more crucial.

Owlets, Apnea Monitors, and So-called SIDS-Preventing Devices

One of the most common Safe to Sleep questions doesn't have anything to do with bed-sharing, swaddling, Back to Sleep, or any AAP guidelines. By the time you read this, chances are you'll already have seen targeted advertising for a supposedly "SIDS-preventing" monitor that promises to trade a few hundred of your hard-earned dollars for complete peace of mind. These expensive devices rely on exploitative marketing and peddle real-life SIDS tragedies for profit. Yet even putting moral outrage aside (shouldn't a SIDS-preventing device be affordable and accessible for all?), I would absolutely support buying any device that saved infant lives.

These don't. There's no science to show that they decrease the risk of SIDS, and pediatricians only see harms with their use. There are more false alarms than protective alerts, leading to worsening fatigue and a circle of never-ending baby checking and anxiety. It's why I don't recommend them to my patients and didn't use one for my daughter. As soon as we find a monitor, machine, mechanism, or miracle that actually reduces the risk of SIDS, I promise I'll be the first to embrace it.

Bed, Bassinet, and Beyond: What's the Deal with Extended Room Sharing?

One thing that makes practicing—and preaching—strict Safe to Sleep guidance is that our AAP handouts can make it seem as if all recommendations are created equal. It's clear from our research that some ingredients to creating a safe-sleep setup (like Back to Sleep and removing tobacco exposure) are extremely important, with no real room for modification. Other SIDS-prevention strategies, however, rest on much shakier data.

Extended room sharing (having your baby sleep in the same room as you for at least six months and up to a year) falls into the not-so-strong-science category. The protective association is weak across studies, and the link is also likely confounded by other factors—like the fact that breastfeeding protects against SIDS and breastfeeding parents tend to room share. It's possible that there is some direct SIDS protection from sleeping in the same room as your baby and allowing your sleep-wake cycles to stay in sync for longer. So I never discourage any parent from attempting extended room sharing if they're willing to give it a try. It's certainly a necessary reality for the first few weeks, where around-the-clock feeding means that going back and forth between your room and baby's will be unsustainable (and make almost any amount of breastfeeding impossible, which we'll discuss in the next chapter). But after four to eight weeks, once breastfeeding is established and/or baby is sleeping at least six hours at a time, the decision to share a room becomes a little less clear-cut. I have seen time and time again (and experienced myself) how, after a few months of having a noisy, restless infant next to your bed, getting a good stretch of sleep (finally!) is almost impossible. And again, we know that interrupted sleep is associated with SIDS. Each family is different, and you'll need to evaluate the reality of your own situation in real time. But if you end up giving your little one an eviction notice, a few weeks (or months) before her six-month birthday, that doesn't mean you've abandoned Safe to Sleep practices altogether.

Safe sleep is a truly nuanced issue but rarely gets the measured, realistic discussion it deserves. Safe to Sleep promoters cite the life-and-death stakes and criticize those of us who even mention "safer bed-sharing" as being cavalier, uncaring, or even medically inappropriate. No way. I take SIDS just as seriously—if not more seriously—than I did before I became a mother. I know you do too, and it's why I'm showing you the full spectrum of research and guidelines behind infant sleep safety. These recommendations are the perfect starting point for a conversation with your pediatrician. Reflect, discuss, plan, and adapt as needed. But above all, know that these guidelines are here so that you can make the best, safest, and most realistic choices for you and your family.

THE BOTTOM LINE

5 out of 5 Pediatrician Parents Agree

- Strict Safe to Sleep in a separate bassinet is still safest in a perfect world; everyone should strive to meet these guidelines, but most parents will have at least one time (and more; likely many more) when this isn't feasible.

- It's safer to practice safer co-sleeping than to fall asleep holding a baby or becoming a sleep-deprived zombie.

- Before baby is born, make two setups: a strict, AAP-blessed Safe to Sleep bassinet and a safer bed-sharing space.

- If you do share your bed with baby, you'll have to follow these basic rules: firm mattress low to the floor; no blankets; no fancy co-sleepers; baby outside mom, not in between parents; no drinking, drugs, or smoking; and Back to Sleep is still the law of the land.

- There aren't any monitors (for now, at least) that prevent SIDS, and the false alarms add needless stress and fatigue.

- Sharing a bedroom with your baby is a logistical feeding necessity for the first four to eight weeks of life. After that, the SIDS-preventing benefits are unclear, so if evicting your tiny roommate to their nursery helps you get more sleep, that's okay.

7

LET'S TALK ABOUT BREAST, BABY

• •

A Slogan-Free Approach to a
Surprisingly Nuanced Topic

The modern parent is nothing if not a planner. Increasing expectations for raising a baby these days means that so much of pregnancy, or however you await your baby's arrival, is spent preparing for what lies ahead. This is true even for breastfeeding, and it seems most parents have already made up their minds about how their baby will get nutrition long before delivery. But for first-time parents, it is almost impossible to understand exactly what this decision entails. The choice is usually binary. Pediatricians meet most parents after delivery either fully committed to exclusive breastfeeding or disinterested in trying. The reality, however, is anything but simple.

This chapter details my unique philosophy, one that truly (and finally!) understands the nuanced approach you should take when deciding if, how, and how much breast milk you plan to give your newborn. As a pediatrician, I'm here to refocus the conversation on *health*—of parents and baby. While the health benefits of breast milk are real and important, it's just as critical to examine how these benefits compare to the stress, discomfort, and even purely logistical challenges that you'll likely face when striving to provide breast milk to your infant.

You see, it used to be simple. Once upon a time, women had magical pregnancies. They danced through the meadows in flowing Grecian gowns and a crown of wildflowers until their exact due date. When they went into labor, they were lifted by a flock of doves and laid onto a fresh bed of lavender. Surrounded by loved ones, they smiled through childbirth and delivered a beautiful baby who was placed on their breast, only to immediately latch and feed on ample, flowing mother's milk. Two rainbows appeared, and there were never any wars or famine again.

Between social media and my own expectations, it was hard for me not to think my breastfeeding journey would be this easy. And my training as a "breast is best" pediatrician certainly didn't help manage these expectations. The "breast is best" campaign, still championed by many pediatricians, has a long and complicated history. Back in Ye Olden Days, babies were breastfed and formula didn't exist. Some babies certainly died if they could not get enough breast milk. Others relied on lactating community members—either voluntarily or by coercion—to provide what they were unable to. People also made their own formulas, which sometimes worked but often weren't safe or able to provide adequate nutrition.

As society and medicine modernized, things changed. In the nineteenth century, two scientific advances collided. In 1810, Nicolas Appert popularized a preservation technique that would be used to create both evaporated and condensed milk, the same technology that is needed to create liquid and powdered formula. Then in 1865, after years of research into the components of breast milk, chemist Justus von Liebig patented the first infant formula specifically engineered to mimic human milk. The market took off, with food companies quickly jumping in to make their own version of this "ideal infant food." By the 1920s, it was common for manufacturers to market directly to doctors—even partnering with the American Medical Association to earn their seals of approval. By the mid-twentieth century, this combination of marketing and medical recommendations had many women ditching breast-feeding altogether. By the early 1970s, over 75% of babies were formula fed, almost all with commercially made products.

While sanitation standards at that time were good enough in the United States to assure that powdered formulas—made with tap water—were generally safe, the same couldn't be said for other countries. Manufacturers quickly turned their eye to the global market, pushing commercial formulas in nations where clean water wasn't always guaranteed. The resulting tragedy—with infants dying from formula made with contaminated water—brought renewed attention to the safety of infant formula.

Sparked by international protests and outrage, the public health community found itself reflecting upon the questions that had been so cleverly swept aside by the baby food companies: Is formula *really* better for babies? Could denying infants breast milk *actually* be causing some harm? This introspection—as well as effective lobbying from religious groups whose pro-breastfeeding advocacy aligned with a vision of traditional domesticity—led to a renewed commitment to studying breastfeeding in earnest. Research began to show that breast milk does have real health benefits, including a lower risk of allergies, diabetes, and obesity. The result was one of the largest course corrections in medical history, with pediatricians around the world quickly cutting ties with their infant formula sponsors and embracing a simple, infamous slogan: "breast is best."

The shift has been long-lasting, and most pediatricians to this day are taught to promote exclusive breastfeeding as the gold standard of infant nutrition. My training was no different. I told parents in the newborn nursery to avoid supplementing with formula, and later during clinic visits had them pump their breasts every three hours until their nipples were raw to try to boost their supplies. I remember one mother asking me permission to please give one formula bottle overnight to her one-month-old infant for an extra three hours of sleep. As a brand-new resident, I was scared to say yes. It pains me to remember hedging my answer, espousing outdated "breast is best" philosophy as I tepidly "allowed" this mother to be less exhausted.

It wasn't my fault, and it isn't the fault of any obstetrician, pediatrician, or other health-care provider whose approach to breastfeeding advice still comes with a heavy, black-and-white dose of "breast is best." There's been progress, for sure. These days, as we learn about the (real!) benefits of breastfeeding, we also learn that there are real medical indications that suggest it's time to supplement with formula. But the basics of how to promote breastfeeding, and the nuances of if, when, and how to use the tools available (including formula) to establish a feeding plan that's best for each family, remain completely absent from our training. It takes years of additional study—and often our own personal experience—to understand the challenges of breastfeeding. The science of helping parents reach their own personal breastfeeding goals is real, but it's sadly not something the majority of pediatricians have the opportunity to learn.

Adherence to a pro-breastfeeding doctrine—without any actual training in the science behind it—is in fact the origin of the "fed is best" countermovement. By the early 2000s, the medical community had applied so much pressure to avoid using formula that some mothers—and even some health-care providers who had been told to promote breastfeeding but not how to recognize when it was failing—stopped giving it to babies who truly needed this additional food and fluids. The tragic result was that several healthy babies, right here in the United States, died from dehydration. The outcry took shape as the "fed is best" movement, based on a simple premise: Parents are encouraged to just feed their baby. It's a message that lives on in today's modified "fed is best" guides. And I get it. "Breast is best" philosophy is ubiquitous and exhausting, with exclusive breastfeeding pressures coming from more sources than ever before. A new world of lactation coaches, naturopaths, bloggers, and chiropractors—all with targeted online advertising—now evangelize exclusive breastfeeding in order to sell their products and services. So many parents, simply exhausted by a barrage of unrealistic expectations, turn to guides that embrace a "fed is best" philosophy that gives them permission to just exist, simply survive, and let their baby do the same.

The thing is, like every part of parenthood, this conversation is much more nuanced than a simple slogan. The key flaw in all these approaches is that they rely on minimizing the very real benefits of breastfeeding. And while I can certainly appreciate—as a mother who struggled deeply with providing breast milk myself—the guilt-free sentiment, misinformation isn't the answer. It's possible to embrace the benefits (and joys!) of breastfeeding while still engaging in a measured, realistic conversation. Telling new parents that breastfeeding can't have benefits, or isn't worth trying, is the same all-or-none approach that takes away agency and even bodily autonomy. Shouldn't parents be able to decide what's right for them based on information that's as honest, complete, and agenda-free as possible?

My own counseling with families embraces open, individualized discussions that prioritize the health of each specific parent-infant pair. It's why, despite my general support of promoting breastfeeding, I advised Amy's mother to stop pumping altogether. Amy had been born a few weeks early and couldn't get the hang of latching on to the breast. Despite weeks of lactation consultant appointments with an expert provider, Amy never managed to stay on the breast. And while her mother pumped every three hours (even setting an alarm overnight to do this), her supply remained low. When I met them, Amy was one month old, and when I asked about breastfeeding, it brought her mother to tears. Struggling with postpartum anxiety, her worries focused sharply on how much breast milk Amy was getting. Why couldn't she provide more than six ounces per day? She had tried pumping more frequently, taken herbal supplements, and read every online post about how to increase her supply. She felt like a failure.

Through more conversation, we were able to work through why she was in fact a "good mother," no matter how much breast milk Amy consumed. I explained that, in this case, I felt strongly that it was better for Amy to get *no* breast milk at all if this would spare her mother needless physical and emotional anguish. I didn't hide any of the positive health effects of breast milk from Amy's mother. In fact, I did the opposite and reviewed them in great detail. But as I went through the science behind each benefit, I explained why it all paled in comparison to the real-life harms we were seeing from obsessive pumping. Attached to a pump, Amy's mother felt distanced from her daughter, and even the most expensive, fancy, hands-free machinery made it harder to snuggle and bond. She hated the feeling of the plastic vacuum sealed to her breast, her nipples cracked and bled, and her sleep was worse than ever. The answer was clear, and I wrote Amy's mother a new prescription: how to wean from pumping and how to refocus on her own mental and physical well-being, by far the most important contributors to her daughter's health.

It is entirely possible to embrace an individualized, flexible approach to breastfeeding and still have it be a "success," no matter how much breast milk your infant consumes. Yes, Amy's mother's weaning was in fact her version of successful breastfeeding, something she happily expressed to me three weeks later as a more-rested mother, better able to engage in her treatment for postpartum anxiety, and much better able to love and enjoy her still-gorgeous, formula-fed bundle of joy. If you follow a few basic principles and seek out the right, reputable resources to support you, your own personalized breastfeeding journey will be successful too.

Set Yourself Up to Be a Breastfeeder

As long as a new parent isn't struggling with some of the medical contraindications and mental health problems that make breastfeeding less beneficial than pure bottle-feeding from the get-go, I always recommend *trying* to breastfeed.

It's becoming an increasingly fun sport to shoot down the science behind breastfeeding, either glossing over the known benefits or denying them completely. But science doesn't care if you insult it; it stays true nonetheless. More studies are needed, but there is plenty of good science to show that breast milk benefits a baby's immune system. Antibodies (such a hot topic these days) are just one of the many bioactive components of a healthy immune system that can be transferred through breast milk. The exact mechanisms are still being studied, but the link is clear. It's been proven that breast milk helps babies fight infections and can help babies have fewer serious illnesses in the first year. We also see lower rates of childhood diseases such as allergies and ear infections later on in children who were breastfed as babies.

Another huge benefit of breast milk—also closely related to immune development—is how it promotes infant intestinal health. So-called good bacteria in a baby's gut do better with breast milk around, which is probably why premature babies are less likely to get serious intestinal infections (called necrotizing enterocolitis) when given breast milk—an association so strong that it's now routine practice for a preemie infant in the NICU to receive donated breast milk whenever a lactating parent's milk doesn't meet feeding demands.

Babies who receive breast milk also have a lower risk of sudden infant death syndrome (SIDS), and there is evidence suggesting that both breastfeeding parents and their babies are protected from certain types of cancer later in life. Cardiovascular disease, diabetes, and other inflammatory conditions have also been shown to happen less in parents who have breastfed their infants.

And it's crucial to understand that breastfeeding *can* be a positive experience. Not only are there health benefits, but the actual process of breastfeeding is often an enjoyable one! I complain constantly about my struggles with providing breast milk for my baby, but the truth is that I liked my actual breastfeeding. It's the pumping I hated.

I gave birth committed to exclusive breastfeeding. My gorgeous milk monster, however, had other plans. For a variety of reasons—including my daughter's jaundice and low sugars, my relatively low milk supply, her prematurity and struggle with latching, my own knowledge gaps in how to promote breastfeeding, and my anxiety and exhaustion requiring the occasional nap during which my husband relied on bottle-feeding—she ended up not ever getting the hang of breastfeeding. Instead, I pumped maniacally to try to give her as much expressed breast milk as possible. On my best day, that was about two thirds of her intake. But even with the fanciest, most expensive, hands-free and portable breast pump, the machinery still created a real emotional and physical distance from my daughter. I hated the feeling of pumping, and my nipples hurt at least a little all the time. At my worst, I compulsively slathered lanolin on my nipples openly at work, even leaving them to air outside of my bra when more understanding coworkers were in the room. And pumping at work in a society that provides no real support for it was emotionally and physically draining. At seven months, I decided to finally let myself stop—and cried needlessly as I weaned off pumping and transitioned to exclusive formula feeding.

My baby did great. Looking back, I wish that I had given myself permission to stop sooner, or at least not have so much unnecessary "bad mom" guilt for weaning. But that's just one story, and my personal breastfeeding journey could have looked very different in different circumstances. What if my daughter and I had been able to establish her latch? If I had had a longer maternity leave, more societal support, had the skills and tools I needed to help my daughter feed mostly at the breast, with pumping as a much-less-frequent inconvenience? There are numerous ways in which the joys of breastfeeding could have outweighed the hassle. And while I regret pushing myself to pump for seven months as an exercise in unnecessary mom-guilt-fueled torture, I don't regret giving breastfeeding an honest try.

In most cases, it makes sense to try to breastfeed. While there's no such thing as Pinterest-perfect breastfeeding with those doves, Grecian robes, and flowering fields, I have in fact spoken to countless mothers who genuinely enjoyed a full year or more of breastfeeding. You deserve the chance for this to be your story, or to create whatever breastfeeding narrative is best for you. Let's be honest about the challenges of breastfeeding reality without resigning parents for whom this is biologically and emotionally possible to not even try. This resignation not only makes it less likely for breastfeeding to be successful—or enjoyable—but deprives you of the chance to experience breastfeeding yourself, and then make the decision if, how much, and for how long to continue based on your own personal journey. Because the truth is that while it's easy to stop breastfeeding (milk dries up!), if you don't give it a solid effort in the beginning, it's challenging to get that milk back.

Even when I was an almost-board-certified pediatrician, I had no real understanding of how maximizing early breastfeeding sets the stage for long-term success, and why this is really the most important reason to do it. I assumed, like so many new parents do, that avoiding formula, pushing through painful latches, and trading sleep for breastfeeding practice was to give babies the most breast milk and the least formula possible during those first, formative weeks of life. While it's true that an increased amount of breast milk will likely provide some increase in those immune and intestinal health benefits we talked about, I hardly even consider this when creating an early infant feeding plan. Instead, I let parents know that the single most important reason to work toward maximum at-the-breast feeding right away is simply to keep your options open. By putting in extra effort early on, you'll maximize the chances that breastfeeding will be a positive and sustainable experience for months to come.

It's simple (if tragically underexplained) biology. Childbirth and the postpartum period are a whirl of hormones, chemicals, physiological changes, and a time of complete flux. There is a finely regulated but highly dynamic biochemical ballet that scientists are learning more and more about each day. After delivery, the dance becomes even more complicated. This is particularly true when it comes to syncing your baby's nutritional needs with your body's ability to meet them (now that your baby is no longer sitting inside you like an adorable parasite with a direct connection to the nutrients in your bloodstream).

It's a tough task, but your (now separated) bodies are smart. The postpartum body quickly kicks into gear with those same hormones (plus some new ones) to rev up a milk supply that is custom-fit to baby's needs. This milk-making internal machinery relies on the biology of hormonal reflex arcs and feedback loops. And parent-infant communication relies on a different science: economics.

It's supply and demand. In order to keep hormone levels high enough to kick off (and build up) milk, breasts need near-constant signaling that reflects exactly how much and how often an infant needs to feed. It's not just about the total amount of nipple stimulation. Longer stretches without a session at the breast (especially in that first week) disrupt hormone levels and make it harder to build a supply even if you "make up" for them with more nursing, hand-expressing, or pumping later in the day. And any time that your infant's feeding and breast stimulation are out of sync, it disrupts the carefully choreographed dance. It's why too much pumping, formula, and bottle-feeding early on can interfere with establishing breastfeeding. They not only create a time when your milk-demand signaling is out of sync, but it's a disconnection that tends to get perpetuated. I've seen (personally and professionally) how pumping "to boost supply" leads to an empty breast when baby is hungry next, leading to a bottle-feed, leading to more pumping, leading to more bottle-feeding—all coming at the cost of practicing a latch, and better boosting milk supply through at-the-breast feeding.

The newborn period is the most critical time for this supply-demand coordination, and sets the stage for the months ahead. It's during the first four to eight weeks that the amount of milk is really established; while it can be boosted a bit after, it's much more challenging and there are diminishing returns on your effort. It's also a key time for establishing a latch. At-the-breast feeding isn't *just* the best way to make sure your baby's cues and your hormone levels stay tightly connected. It's also, almost universally, a more enjoyable experience than pumping and makes months of breastfeeding sustainable.

Nothing is black-and-white. There's a good chance you'll use formula, a bottle of expressed milk, or somehow modify this all-day nursing buffet to meet your specific postpartum needs. It's not irrevocable, and introducing formula does *not* ruin your chances of exclusive or maximal breastfeeding. Understanding this biology, however, does help demystify why strategies that maximize nursing and minimize bottles and pumping lead to increased, sustained breastfeeding. In the end, you can use this guide to simply do your best, customizing your approach to meet your individual emotional and physical needs. By giving it the college try, you'll be able to provide the best, maximal amount of breast milk specifically for you and your infant (even if that amount ends up being part or none of their milk intake!). Here are the pediatrician-mom approved, biologically sound ways to give breastfeeding an honest effort, setting you up for long-term success on your breastfeeding journey, whatever it looks like.

Be Prepared

As is so often the case in life, knowing what to expect is half of the breastfeeding battle (and yes, it will likely feel like a battle sometimes!). We've talked about just how dynamic the process of breastfeeding is, and it's an ever-changing adventure filled with learning, laughs, tears, heartbreak, and triumph. Breastfeeding doesn't have to be miserable, but it's rarely an easy experience. Chances are that it will take some time for you and your milk-monster to get into a groove that feels right to you both.

You should expect it to take work, but know that any bumps along the way are in no way a reflection of your parenting, or a reflection on what your breastfeeding journey will look like going forward. If you can, try to familiarize yourself with some of the basics before your little one arrives. Whether it's a breastfeeding class, educational videos, or chatting with seasoned breastfeeders to get some tips and tricks, it'll be helpful to practice some simple positioning techniques and learn more about the mechanics.

It's also important to know that the initial struggles with breastfeeding are likely temporary, or at the very least should improve with time. There's no need to endure excruciating pain even in those first few weeks. But few parents realize that the majority of serious physical discomfort—and the real burden of around-the-clock, at-the-breast feeding—gets better. Understanding that this isn't forever will help you frame just how much you are able to tolerate.

A.B.N. (Always Be Naked)

One of my favorite memories from my residency was when I walked into a patient's room while on an overnight emergency room shift and found her mother standing topless, idly scrolling on her phone while her infant slept in her crib. As I apologized for barging in and offered to come back later, she laughed, shrugged, and told me to come on in. "I'm a nursing mom, I'm always topless. This won't look any different next time you come around."

"Always topless" quickly became my milk-making motto. By the time you finish with an at-the-breast feed, lather your nipples in whatever ointment provides some relief, put your nursing bra and clothes back on, then sit down for a minute of fully clothed repose, it'll probably be time for your next feed. And keeping your breasts open-to-air is also the best defense against nipple irritation, an added bonus to postpartum exhibitionism.

Most important, staying naked (or mostly naked, most of the time) means making skin-to-skin and newborn nipple exploration the norm. In the first week especially, establishing breastfeeding isn't about creating a feeding schedule that meets your baby's hunger needs. Your baby will be born with a stomach that's literally the size of a pea. They also will lose some uterine hot-tub water weight in the first week, and pediatricians aren't looking to make them chunky quite yet. We have lots of ways to know that they're getting enough colostrum (until your milk comes in, usually around three to five days) to stay hydrated, maintain their blood sugar, and keep jaundice at bay. So as long as those things are going well, you really don't have to worry about the exact amount of milk making it into your newborn's teeny tiny stomach. Instead, those first few days are about practicing latching, stimulating your nipple, and letting your bodies synchronize.

Maximizing toplessness also makes it easy to keep feeding (or at least feeding practice) a frequent occurrence. Feeding and stimulating your breast at least every three hours, ideally by having your baby directly stretching your nipple with their mouth, is important to establishing those hormonal reflex arcs. Cluster feeding—when babies seem to feed almost constantly for hours at a time, usually in the evening—is common. It's related to their in-utero day/night reversal, and if you're able to indulge it, your supply and latch will build more quickly.

Be Judicious with Breast Pump and Paci Use

In Chapter 11 we'll dive into detail about the myths that inform the binky ban, and why I don't think making pacis strictly verboten is the way to go. But being mindful makes a lot of sense. "Nipple confusion" is nonsense—babies are smart and can tell nipples apart just fine, they just usually prefer milk from a fast-flowing bottle over straight-from-the-tap breast milk they have to work harder for. But if you're using a pacifier to soothe a hungry baby rather than taking that opportunity to practice nursing, it makes sense that this would interfere with your breastfeeding journey. I absolutely used possibly SIDS-preventing plastic pacification right away, and I'd do it again despite all my breastfeeding struggles. I would just remember to be judicious in how I used it. I advise parents to save their pacifiers, as much as possible, for after a feed, using them primarily once their little one is swaddled and placed in their bassinet. If it falls out, let it stay out. It's an important tool for soothing and sleeping, but nothing that should replace at-the-breast exploration or be forced into your baby's calm, closed mouth.

It also makes sense to be judicious with your breast pump use early on. There's nothing "bad" about pumping, but as we discussed, it's likely to interfere with your body's ability to respond to your baby's erratic, unpredictable feeding schedule. Once a latch is established, you shouldn't have to pump for the first month. I wish I had known this, and like so many, I falsely assumed that early, frequent pumping was the key to breastfeeding success. Yes, there will be times when early pumping makes sense. If your baby struggles to latch, has a painful latch, or if you feel in any way that mechanical milk expression will provide you comfort, that's totally fine. Just chat with your lactation consultant so you can strategize and customize. Sometimes small amounts of hand expression can provide enough relief for aching breasts and minimize the use of pumping, and other times a small amount of bottle feeding will calm a "hangry" baby enough to let them practice their latch in earnest. And sometimes pumping is inevitable, at least temporarily. It's legitimately complicated, and the reason that expert, certified, medically trained lactation consultants exist. Find yours (even if that means searching online for a telehealth visit!) and make sure you get the support you need in making the best pumping choices for you and your baby.

Even if you're able to postpone pumping until your baby's one-month birthday, you should still have a breast pump at home before your baby is born. In the United States, these are covered by all insurances, so make sure your OB has been able to hook you up. Like with breastfeeding, you'll want to learn how it works and get familiar with the parts. Talk to your OB or lactation consultant if available (bring your pump into one of your visits!), watch videos, chat with other pumping parents, and give yourself a chance to ask questions and get to know this piece of milk-making machinery.

Bottles and Formula Have a Role in Many Cases— You Just Need to Be Mindful

Let's continue the theme. You may very well need to bring bottles—with formula or breast milk—into the equation during the first weeks of your little one's life. There are lots of times when a baby's medical needs mean that some amount of formula is the way to go. And there are even more times when your own postpartum needs make bottle feeding a truly beneficial intervention. I know that my own struggles fall into this category. With my anxiety, emerging depression, sleep deprivation, and intense C-section pain, the ability to use formula feeds to get more sleep was a godsend. So if your own needs— even just wanting a little more rest or needing a break from the constant breastfeeding song and dance—bring formula into the equation, that's okay. Get rest, feel confident in your decision, and move on. You'll reassess after your nap and decide if prioritizing at-the-breast feeding still makes sense, how much effort is possible, and what resources you can use to meet your new-and-improved custom breastfeeding goals.

Safe Sleep Practices Make It Harder to Breastfeed

Yup, I said it. It is a truth universally (and sadly) unacknowledged that bed-sharing makes breastfeeding much, much easier. Sleeping next to an infant gives them all-night access to at-the-breast snacking, helping both of you establish your latch and increase your supply. And it's much more sustainable than the breastfeeding, solo-sleeping parent's ritual of waking up, undressing, unswaddling, latching, swaddling, placing back to sleep, then getting back into bed.

While this is the main reason that evangelical lactation organizations push bed-sharing and overstate its safety, it doesn't mean that it's enough reason to abandon Safe to Sleep practices altogether! I stand by my "Co-sleep No More" guidelines, encouraging you to give by-the-book safe sleep a real try while preparing for harm-reduced bed-sharing plan B. It's just important to understand that this is a calculated trade-off, meaning that pediatricians are asking you to make breastfeeding harder in order to make sleep safer. The science, of course, is evolving, and I truly hope that we can find a way to maximize sleep safety and optimize breastfeeding simultaneously. But for now, remember that we've stacked the deck a little bit against you, and if your baby gets less breast milk because of it, that's not your fault.

Not Everyone Will Have the Same Ease with Breastfeeding

There are countless reasons that you and your baby might have a much more challenging time establishing breastfeeding, or even not be able to establish sustainable breastfeeding at all. In the bad old days, pediatricians used to say that fewer than 5% of women had a "real, medical" reason they didn't produce enough milk for their little ones. But breastfeeding science disagrees, and the elaborate ballet of supply and demand relies on more factors than even the experts understand (at least yet!). Potential obstacles include having had a C-section, infertility, and dozens of underlying health conditions (like thyroid disease, postpartum depression, polycystic ovarian syndrome, the list goes on). When you add in the logistical, societal, and emotional struggles that new parents face when trying to breastfeed, you start to wonder how anyone makes enough milk at all!

Focus on getting the medical and mental health care you need. Optimizing your own health is more important than any amount of breast milk your baby gets—and it's also the best way to maximize the chances that your baby gets more breast milk! Another win-win.

It's Completely Okay If It Doesn't Work Out Perfectly—or Even At All

We have to embrace that the health benefits of breastfeeding only matter when they are compared to what the actual experience of breastfeeding is like for a parent and baby. The barriers to breastfeeding are super real and super challenging: Supply issues, difficult latch, workplaces that don't support pumping, inadequate parental leave, and insufficient long-term lactation support all make it hard for even the most determined among us to exclusively breastfeed. If it doesn't work out—like even a little, not one drop of breast milk—it will be *completely* fine.

It's exactly what I told Charlie's dads when they reached out to me for some new-baby advice. Having finalized the adoption paperwork, their nursery was all set and they were eager to create a feeding plan that would assure their precious daughter had the best nutrition possible. There were places, they told me, where breast milk could be purchased online. Was this safe? Would a nursing mom friend be willing to share? Was *just* giving formula (*gasp*) actually okay? I assured them that any formula would be perfect. Searching the dark web for "liquid gold" was unnecessary. The fact that they were thinking so carefully about their daughter's feeding plan meant that she would be not only nourished, but truly loved and attended to.

And for biological parents, my advice is often similar. I've helped plenty of mothers without partners, with peripartum depression, with unsupportive partners, with little parental leave, with unsupportive work environments, with limited financial resources (portable pumps and lactation consultants are more expensive than subsidized or bulk formula!), or who are just simply overwhelmed with breastfeeding, or say "no" altogether to breastfeeding. The breastfeeding conversation too often is tied to privilege, speaking only to biological, partnered parents with the time, money, and support needed for breastfeeding benefits to consistently outweigh its burden. In many situations, providing breast milk *isn't always* a reasonable option—but when it is, it is in fact worth a try.

Deciding If/How Much/How Long to Continue Breastfeeding Is a Personal Decision

Sometimes, breastfeeding goes great. Sometimes, it's clear that breastfeeding just isn't working. Most of the time, it's a much more complicated equation. My later struggles aligned more with Amy's mother (whom we met earlier in this chapter), trying to balance the benefits of giving breast milk to my baby with the agonies of pumping. But there are countless, varying examples of how the risks and benefits of breastfeeding stack up for each individual. One of my colleagues, for example, was a talented and passionate breastfeeder of her children, so it was the logistics of pumping at work to maintain her supply that made the decision to introduce some formula (and decrease stressful pump breaks) a favorable one. Another finally fought against breast milk–only pressures when she saw how replacing an overnight feeding session with a bottle led to an extra block of uninterrupted sleep that completely changed her ability to function.

Your breastfeeding goals are yours. You are smart, capable, and fully able to decide what aspects of breastfeeding are important, how important they are, which strategies are worthwhile to get you there, and which physical limitations simply make exclusively breastfeeding unreasonable. You also deserve counseling that understands your specific goals, embracing just how valid they are and what they're based on.

We are only now just starting to pay attention to the deep disparities in breastfeeding across different groups, and reckon with our own role in perpetuating them. There is a tremendous amount of racial and cultural bias that comes into play when we health-care professionals provide breastfeeding guidance. Just like "breast is best" stemmed from the assumption that all parents were shoving unnecessary, medically marketed formula in their babies' mouths, "fed is best" assumes that these same (mostly white, often affluent) parents are at their wits' ends and need permission to stop breastfeeding.

I'm guilty of it myself. It's hard not to project my own breastfeeding turmoil onto others and assume that everyone I counsel has pushed themself too hard to breastfeed, wants permission to just give formula, and has a social network that ascribes to the same "breast is best"–style preaching that mine does. But breastfeeding pressures are different across communities, and there are plenty of cultural and religious factors that can positively or negatively impact a person's perception of breastfeeding. If we want to promote breastfeeding support that truly honors an individual's well-being, we'll have to dig deep. And this absolutely means acknowledging—and hopefully reckoning with—the centuries of structural racism, systemic inequality, and intergenerational trauma that inform the modern breastfeeding experience we see today.

The history of breastfeeding is much more complicated, and even more tragic, than the horror stories that sparked the "breast is best" and "fed is best" portray. For example, it wasn't too long ago in the United States that enslaved Black mothers were routinely robbed of the right to control their own bodies in countless ways, including nursing their own children—and were instead forced to serve as "wet nurses" for the children of slave owners. The ripple effects were endless, informed by the decades that followed, which saw an ongoing oppression of Black parents (and other marginalized communities). There's no straight line, no simple narrative that explains how we got to where we are today. But there is a notable disparity between feeding practices in this country, with oppressed communities still breastfeeding much less on average. To say it's complicated is an understatement, and my favorite modern breastfeeding researchers spend their careers dissecting the complex interplay between culture, race, religion, socioeconomic status, social supports, community psychology, medical messaging, and how these impact breastfeeding practices in different groups.

While you don't have to conduct your own PhD research into this truly fascinating topic, you should know that your own relationship with breastfeeding may be just as messy—and that's okay. And you should also feel free to demand the type of thoughtful counseling that understands this. One-size-fits-all advice is never the right approach, and it fails to understand what new parents are bringing to the table. "Breast is best" misses the mark when it puts undue pressure on parents who are determined to maximize their supply at all costs. It also fails because it assumes that the desire to breastfeed is universal, untainted, divorced from historical oppression. "Fed is best" deprives those same, perfectionist parents (yes, like me!) from true bodily autonomy, replacing the supports that would optimize the breastfeeding experience with a glib "it doesn't matter." And it also fails parents who come from communities where breastfeeding is discouraged—something that happens for many reasons, including the legacy of coerced breastfeeding we are just finally starting to discuss.

Use (or Ditch) Whatever Breastfeeding Supports You Can Find—but Stay Clear of a Few "Red Flag" Options

If and when breastfeeding struggles emerge, the most important thing is remembering that you don't have to deal with it alone. Instead, you too can find a seasoned, certified expert to help you steer your breastfeeding ship. It's something that's increasingly available to parents around the country (thank you, tele-lactation appointments!). And this consultant will partner with your pediatrician to see what additional supports make sense (like when tongue tie should be evaluated by a reputable ENT surgeon, or when physical therapy for torticollis is an actual, medical need). Sticking to these lactation gurus will assure that you don't get caught up in the for-profit breastfeeding hype, and let you reach the personal, scientifically sound breastfeeding goals of your wildest dreams.

It really is hard to navigate it alone, especially in today's world of for-profit breastfeeding marketing. Online, parents find endless products and services that claim to be strict necessities for any baby's breastfeeding success. And while I am certainly no fan of two-hundred-dollar out-of-pocket, untested therapies, it's okay to consider some of the less-studied options if they're something you want to explore. I know plenty of parents who swear by gentle craniosacral therapy, infant massage, and other similar practices with low risk for harm. Just remember the limitations and keep your expectations in check. These modalities are unregulated, unproven, and performed with high variability. There's no way to know if they'll help any more than a tincture of time, some hands-on latch support, and a therapeutic dose of compassionate listening. As we'll discuss in Chapter 20, reasonably safe interventions that lack science are fine to try—just use some common sense. Reflect on if there's a problem that needs fixing, talk to a real expert, and stay skeptical as you explore the world of for-profit lactation support.

I didn't understand the scope of the pro-breastfeeding madness until I learned from friends and patients the sheer lengths that they've gone to make their breastfeeding a "success." Parents are pushed to try high-velocity chiropractic manipulation, an unproven, unregulated practice with shaky scientific reasoning and no supporting evidence in adults, let alone babies. And in this case, it's not just wasted time and money: Messing around with a baby's spinal cord can (of course!) even be fatal.

And a surgery is a surgery, even if a dentist, chiropractor, naturopath, or unlicensed lactation adviser has sent you there. There's a lot of emerging evidence to show that pediatricians have been correcting tongue ties more than we need to, making us more judicious in when we recommend them than we used to be. Anatomical issues are real, and seasoned pediatricians and ENT doctors will be able to assess when fixing them is likely to help with breastfeeding. It's a medical procedure, with risks and benefits, and a decision we should be thoughtful in making.

Letting an evidence-based lactation expert take the reins is the best way to tune out the noise and only explore the services that make sense for you and your baby. I remember when one mother told me that when she was referred to a locally renowned oral surgeon specializing in tongue ties for her baby's mild latch issues, he explained her baby not only had a terrible tongue and upper lip tie (diagnoses that studies are now showing are rarely problematic), but that he also had a "buccal tie." When I heard this, my jaw almost hit the floor (no pun intended). "Buccal" mucosae are just the inner cheeks, meaning this doctor was suggesting that the baby's cheeks were too strongly connected to his jaw. It doesn't take a pediatrician to realize that baby cheeks—just like those of all humans—are best left firmly attached to one's face.

It took someone trying to sell a quick, expensive "fix" to make this mom reflect and reassess if there really was a problem with her baby's breastfeeding—and what that problem even was. Transitioning her care to a seasoned, certified lactation consultant with a background in evidence-based breastfeeding medicine (they exist!) was a complete game changer. Working together with this lactation expert, her pediatrician, and engaging in some good old reflection on her breastfeeding goals led this mother to an entirely different conclusion. Formula wasn't the enemy. Supplementing allowed her to still provide most nutrition through at-the-breast feeding (which became more comfortable with some simple lactation-counselor-approved positioning strategies), and with time, she was even able to increase the amount of breast milk her baby received—no risky laser procedures necessary.

The reality is that anyone selling breastfeeding as an extreme sport is more interested in making money than helping mothers and babies. Breastfeeding is important, and helping you reach your breastfeeding goals is a worthy endeavor. But it isn't the be-all and end-all of parenting. If someone makes you feel that maximizing the amount of breast milk your baby consumes is worth pursuing at all costs, it makes sense to take a step back and question their motives.

In the end, I promise you that whatever amount of breastfeeding you can and want to do is better than fine, as long as it's what *you* want to do. There's no magical amount of breast milk—or even formula—that will guarantee health and happiness. The most important thing is to make sure you're making feeding decisions that are truly *yours*. For most of you, this means embracing some pretty simple advice: try breastfeeding, breastfeed as much as you can, and give as much formula as you need to keep the excess stress at bay—if and when it starts to creep in. If your baby's belly is full and your milk supply is active, you are, by definition, a successful breastfeeder, no matter how much formula it takes to keep you there. And when breastfeeding becomes too much for you even with formula in the mix, just stop. The American Academy of Pediatrics recommends exclusively breastfeeding through the first year, an arbitrary goal that sets the majority of parents up for unnecessary "failure." Focus on putting in the effort in the beginning, making sustainable, longer-term breastfeeding more likely, and let the chips fall where they may. Breastfeeding is worth trying in earnest, and something you should continue to do as long as it works for you.

THE BOTTOM LINE

5 out of 5 Pediatrician Parents Agree

- If you can, set yourself up to be a breastfeeder—breastfeeding has real medical benefits and can (eventually) be an enjoyable experience.

- If breastfeeding doesn't work out, that's totally fine and your baby will be healthy and happy.

- It's not all or none—giving formula doesn't mean breastfeeding is a "failure" or that you have to stop giving whatever amount of breast milk you want to.

- The "right" amount of breast milk to give is what works for your preference, lifestyle, and individual choice.

- There are some red flags, though: anyone pushing surgeries, supplements, expensive sessions, or other products without a truly thoughtful, individualized discussion of your breastfeeding goals is selling something and doesn't have your best interests at heart.

8

I LOVE YOU, PLEASE BE QUIET

• •

Dealing with Colic, Reflux,
and Baby Fuss

As a new parent, there's nothing more frustrating than hearing that your infant's daily routine of screaming bloody murder is actually "normal." Who wouldn't think that a pediatrician's description of an inconsolable baby as "healthy" is insane? I have yet to meet a parent who doesn't find themselves, at some point, desperately wondering if their baby's extreme fussiness is cause for alarm. With years of experience caring for colicky, refluxy, and fussy kids in the office, emergency room, and even in the hospital, I'm here to demystify the many causes—both explainable and bewildering—that so often make otherwise perfect babies lose their minds.

There are three main diagnoses: colic, reflux, and formula intolerance. And while the internet will have you believe that all of these are equivalent problems with easy (and expensive) fixes, let's go through the real, scientific, and safe techniques that you should use instead.

Colic

I'll never forget the first time baby Eve came into my office. Even though I was still in the first months of residency and my patient load was light, the fast-paced clinic schedule had me running from room to room. I grabbed Eve's file and looked at her vital signs—all normal for her age. She was here for a "sick visit," and next to "chief complaint," the medical assistant had written "fussiness." I rolled my eyes. Who on earth would bring their child into a doctor for being a fussy baby?

After introducing myself to Eve's parents, I kept my best bedside manner as I listened to their "complaint." Eve was one month old, growing well, eating well, and doing all the normal baby things she should be doing. But she wouldn't stop crying. My training as a medical student had provided me with some basic knowledge that helped guide my questions. On any test, a baby between the ages of three weeks and three months of age who cried for hours at night but had no other problems had "colic." The answer choice for treatment was: don't worry. That baby is fine, move on to more important medical decision-making and go save some babies' lives.

The thing about medical school tests, however, is that you don't take them with a real family sitting in front of you. As Eve's mother detailed her evening routine of rocking a screaming baby who seemed completely miserable, she herself began to break down in tears. She felt so terrible for Eve, she said, why was she so unhappy? And, she could barely admit it, but both parents were miserable, too. No one had slept in days. She just wanted it to stop—not just for Eve, but for everyone. Was she even ready to be a mother? She felt so guilty that she had even thought that, let alone said it out loud to a pediatrician. The tears came more quickly.

I sympathized deeply with Eve's parents, but of course didn't truly begin to understand their experience until I became a mother myself. When my baby was about one month old, I felt that I was just barely getting the hang of things when one winter afternoon, I awoke from a quick nap to the loudest baby screams I had ever heard. I ran, picked up my baby, unswaddled her, rocked her, fed her. She calmed a little but went right back to crying. I swaddled her, swayed, shushed, danced. The crying continued. Maternal and pediatrician anxiety swirled together in my sleep-deprived brain. Try though I might, I couldn't resist unswaddling her, grabbing my stethoscope, and performing a full physical. Her neurological, heart, lung, abdominal, skin examinations were all normal. I looked for the favorite test question answer when a screaming baby does not have just "colic"—a piece of hair wrapped around a baby's toe or finger and causing pain—and found nothing. An hour later, her cries still came and went. I called my best pediatrician friends and presented her case. Everyone agreed: My daughter was okay. Yet even with this additional reassurance, it was hard to shake the feeling that something could be wrong.

So, what *is* colic? There are no fancy lab tests to diagnose it; instead, modern pediatricians rely on symptoms—namely, patterns of crying. The organization the Period of PURPLE Crying coined the mnemonic PURPLE to explain that a baby with colic demonstrates three or more of the following signs:

- **P**—crying that *peaks* when they are around 2 months old
- **U**—crying that is *unexpected* and can come and go without any apparent reason
- **R**—crying that *resists* soothing
- **P**—a look indicating that the baby is in *pain* when they cry
- **L**—crying that can last a *long* time, up to five hours each day
- **E**—crying that usually happens most in the late afternoon and *evening*

My daughter had "colic" like she had read a pediatric text-book. Every evening she would begin crying suddenly and would calm down only intermittently for the next three hours. It was mostly through trial and error that I found a temporary solution. I held her facing outward, my arms wrapped behind her knees so they came up to her belly and her bottom sagged down, as we danced around our living room. I sang along to Top 40 songs and nineties hip-hop playlists, and made up my own music and lyrics during commercial breaks. (To this day, I find myself humming "Mommy and baby are gonna be okay, I know you'll stop crying for no reason one day," one of my catchier original jingles.) Just like Eve's mother, I cried too. I had gone back to work part-time at six weeks, and I still winced in pain as my baby pressed down on my C-section incision site. I was emotionally and physically drained. Hearing that this was "normal" would have only amplified my tears.

Months later, my daughter's fits of colic stopped as suddenly as they had started. As she developed into an exceedingly calm, happy, and "easy" baby, memories of our screaming evening ballet quickly faded. But my experience left me with an entirely new perspective, and I promised to take colic-induced parental stress even more seriously. Too often, I see parents seek the depths of internet misinformation for answers when they feel that modern medicine has dismissed colic as "normal." Babies with colic are *healthy* and *safe*, but you don't have to accept excessive parental suffering. For most families, some strategic tag teaming, decreasing light and noises in the home, and focusing on your *own* self-care are the most success-ful remedies. Once you and your pediatrician agree that colic is the cause of your baby's a capella horror-movie soundtrack, these are the first things to try (and there are plenty of great resources on how to do this, including that same Period of Purple Crying website).

But there are cases when a baby's colicky screaming is just too much for everyone to handle. While the definitive cause of colic remains elusive—most evidence points toward differ-ences in the "good" bacteria, hormones, and other changes in some babies' intestines—there is plenty of data available that guides safe and effective solutions. Let's channel the science we *do* have—along with a hefty dose of common sense—to give you some options that are safe and effective.

We can start by crossing some definite "nos" off the list. These include drops that work to fight the cramp-inducing gut hormones we know are elevated in colicky babies. Drops with ingredients like hyoscine, scopolamine, and dicyclomine make these babies cry less—but don't work any better than reducing light and noise in the home. They also have real side effects, including constipation, sleepiness, and even serious breathing problems. Another "no" is baby acupuncture, which researchers in Norway have found makes babies cry *more*.

Some other remedies are probably safe, but it's still unclear if they work. Newer science suggests that probiotics might be helpful. In Italy, researchers have shown in several studies that using certain lactobacillus probiotic supplements does seem to help babies with symptoms of colic. So, while there's more research to be done, trying a well-regulated infant probiotic drop is one option to keep in your back pocket (and in discussion with your pediatrician, of course).

Another option for addressing serious colic is changing a baby's milk menu. One study by Swedish researchers showed that when sixty breastfeeding women removed cow's milk from their diets, half of them had babies whose colic disappeared, and then reappeared when they reintroduced it. Dozens of well-designed studies since have found similar results. Some have even suggested more restrictive dietary changes may be helpful. An Australian study found that moms who removed cow's milk, nuts, wheat, soy, and fish also saw less crying in their colicky infants.

Of course, there are other practical concerns to weigh here. For example, is taking away your ice cream and pizza going to cause more stress than a screaming (but completely safe and healthy) baby? And what about the medical risks of these diets? In a world with rising rates of serious, life-threatening food allergies—where early introduction of those allergy-inducing foods is a main established prevention technique—an unnecessarily restricted diet could have serious, long-term consequences. Although the initial research on removing nuts, wheat, soy, and fish is compelling, there's not enough consistent data *yet* to outweigh the risks of missing out on early introduction of these awesome allergens in most cases.

I know firsthand how miserable colic can be. So while I'm not going to say it's *never* okay to try a restrictive diet to treat colic, it usually makes sense to try some other sanity-preserving techniques first. And if that doesn't work, and your pediatrician is on board, removing cow's milk is fine to try. Just remember that this isn't the same as saying your baby has a milk "allergy" or even "intolerance." Instead, elimination diets in this case are simply an option for your toolbox, a way to empower you as a parent to use the information that we have and to decide which strategies have the right risk-and-benefit profile to be worth trying. And remember, it's always a decision that you make for a moment in time. You can stop as soon as it stops working for you. If you and your baby plan on consuming cow's milk for preference, nutrition, or even convenience at some point in the future, remember to chat with your pediatrician about a plan for reintroducing it (often around four to six months, when peak colic days have passed) to decrease the risk of developing an allergy later in life.

I know firsthand that when colic hits, parents are at their sleep-deprived wits' end. It's all too easy to be seduced by unregulated products that at best are a waste of money and at worst can cause real harm. You can rest assured that your screaming baby is indeed healthy and safe. But when maximizing your home's chill vibes aren't enough, you can still choose science over salesmen. This isn't the same as giving up—there are real, doctor-approved ways that they can help your baby (and you!) through this terrible newborn rite of passage.

Reflux

Let's dive into baby "reflux," a popular buzzword with "mommy blogs" and pediatricians alike, and one of the most common causes of unnecessary angst and confusion. Reflux is a simpler diagnosis than colic. Babies drink milk through their mouths just like we do, it goes down their esophagus just like our food does, and then enters the stomach through a magical door called the lower esophageal sphincter (LES). The LES—like all sphincters—is just a pressure-operated valve. Our bodies open it when food knocks to get into the stomach, then (ideally) closes it so it doesn't come back up. In grown-ups, there are a lot of things that can make this one-way mechanism go faulty and let stomach juice back up into the esophagus. Stomach juice is acidic, and this hurts, so we call this *heartburn* or *acid reflux*. It's a common, treatable problem that has made the makers of Prilosec, Pepcid, and Tums very, very rich.

As you might have guessed, like almost every part of their bodies, little baby food pipes are different from older kids' and adults'. Their adorable LESes are immature and don't always remember to keep that door shut when food isn't trying to get in. Fortunately, babies drink milk, have less acid in their stomach to begin with, and it's rare for this normal "reflux" to cause significant pain. Instead, it makes babies vomit. Like, almost all babies. By one month of age, half of babies routinely vomit after eating, and by two months, this number increases to 80%. But it goes away. By seven months, only 6% of babies have daily spit-ups, and by their first birthday the rate of routine vomiting is negligible.

Reflux is *normal*. Pediatricians are so unconcerned that we lovingly call these adorable pukers "happy spitters." I'm barely joking when I tell parents that it's the babies who *don't* spit up that worry me. Spit-up only becomes a problem when it makes a baby unhappy. In these cases, we no longer call it "reflux" but GERD (gastroesophageal reflux disease). The most common signs of GERD are stunted growth (if vomiting is severe enough to stop milk from getting digested) and frequent irritability after feeds (because there is so much acid that it becomes painful). This feed-related fussiness is what makes it easy to confuse GERD with colic. The good news is that you don't have to decide this on your own. A seasoned, up-to-date pediatrician will work through all the data you have and decide which diagnosis (if any) makes more sense. Knowing that these are distinct diagnoses—each with different management options—will keep you savvy, letting you work with your pediatrician to create thoughtful and appropriate treatment plans.

What *are* the treatment options if a baby truly has GERD? The most effective method is just giving smaller amounts of milk at a time and holding babies upright for longer than usual after they feed. Let gravity do the work. Elevating babies' heads for sleep, or positioning them on an incline, doesn't help, and is simply an unnecessary obstacle to achieving the safest sleep practices possible. Other remedies—like thickening feeds with rice cereal or commercially sold "thickeners"—don't really work, and they can have side effects like gut infections, especially in premature babies. Yet I still see recommendations for thickened feeds all over the place despite a compelling lack of evidence. One online parenting expert explained to me that while she wasn't aware of any supporting data, she still suggests parents try this approach. Her reasoning: Parents need to feel like they can do something to help their babies spit up less, and thickening milk is a harmless enough option. I disagree. Parents, you're smart. We should all give you the credit you deserve.

By now you might notice some of those themes I promised in my introduction emerging. If your baby is growing and not having frequent lung infections (a very rare effect of severe GERD), there's no one-size-fits-all answer about if, when, and how to start treatment. I'll give you the range of safe and effective options, which should all be discussed with a pediatrician who's had the chance to take a good look at your adorable puking bundle of joy. I frequently see how unnecessary treatments—even those with minimal or rare side effects—just create stress and make parents think their healthy babies have problems that don't really exist. Like colic, it's important to remember that while it's true that your baby is more or less "fine" and not in any danger of serious harm, there are scientifically sound coping strategies that you'll be able to use.

Bookmark this page and do your best to avoid the world of anxiety-inducing, sometimes dangerous online advice.

If simple interventions like giving smaller amounts of milk at a time and holding babies upright for longer than usual after they feed aren't enough, there's still hope. The next step is asking your pediatrician if eliminating cow's milk from a breastfeeding parent's diet (and/or using a special formula without cow's milk if your baby takes any formula) makes sense. It's not because getting rid of cow's milk treats GERD, which is a very common misconception that's prevalent among parents and novice pediatricians alike. It instead, intuitively, treats something called cow's milk protein intolerance. This is a different disease than GERD, with a different cause—some babies' intestines can't digest cow's milk, and the proteins cause inflammation in their gut. While this can cause other symptoms like blood in their poop, it can also just present as fussiness with feeds, vomiting, and weight loss.

Since these are also common symptoms of GERD, pediatricians are now realizing that a good number of babies with "GERD" who don't do better with smaller, upright feedings instead have cow's milk protein intolerance. Luckily, there's an easy way to test which babies fall into which category. Pediatricians work with parents to help them remove all cow's milk from a baby's diet for a few weeks. If your baby gets better, the culprit is cow's milk, so diagnosis and treatment are complete. If your baby doesn't get better, the most likely diagnosis is severe GERD, and that's when it makes sense to give an acid-stopping medicine. We try to use these medicines less than we used to, since it's now known that acid medicines (like Zantac) may make a baby more likely to develop allergies later in life (and have a few other rare side effects if used for many months). But they are still the most effective way to treat serious, real GERD. If a baby has severe, classic GERD that just won't go away, I still use those medications in my practice. In the end, most "reflux" is normal, and true GERD is rare and overtreated. But if it's bothering your baby, it's a problem we can fix.

Formula Intolerance

The last baby-fuss-diagnosis I'll dive into is formula intolerance. First, it's important to understand that when pediatricians talk about "intolerance," we are referring to a real disease called "milk protein intolerance," where a baby's gut struggles so much with cow's milk that there is true inflammation. As I explained above, if a baby has blood in their poop, won't grow, or has pain with eating that doesn't go away with giving smaller, upright feeds, trying specialized formulas and changing a breastfeeding parent's diet are absolutely the way to go. But do fancy formulas help fussy babies even if they *don't* have milk protein intolerance? These days, more and more parents agonize over which special formula is best, with blogs, social media groups, and word-of-mouth rumors convincing them that specific, expensive formulas can create happier, healthier babies.

Does science support this? No—or at least not yet. Yes, we know that for milk protein intolerance and firmly diagnosed colic, elimination diets and hydrolyzed formulas play a role. But for your everyday baby fuss, all the evidence shows that any formula is as good as the next, and that there's absolutely no need to have a breastfeeding parent restrict their diet.

It's not just hydrolyzed formulas and elimination diets that are needlessly stressful. The rapidly expanding market of formulas leaves parents with endless options, and each type is marketed as filling a specific and important need. Formula shoppers will find brands that promise to fix reflux, cure colic, end constipation, promote digestion, or even provide a plant-based source of nutrition proposed to have proven infant health benefits. The science is evolving, and the claims are hard to sort through. Does using lactose as a primary carbohydrate—which has a relatively low glycemic index— really make formula easier to digest? How important is the whey to casein ratio in human babies? Does using organic cow's milk have meaningful environmental and health benefits? What's the perfect amount of DHA to add? Do all babies need probiotics?

We don't have definitive answers to any of these questions yet, with data coming primarily from animal models in the lab, studies conducted by the formula companies themselves, and a whole lot of anecdotal evidence from pediatricians and parents. It means that these formulas—as long as they meet the safety and storage standards of the country they're sold in—are usually fine, and it's very possible a baby might have a nonstandard formula preference. There's just no way to predict which flavor profile will work best for each baby, and there isn't enough science (yet) to say that any fancy formulas are inherently better than the cheapest, generic equivalent of Enfamil or Similac.

A quick caveat: As modern scientists, pediatricians are happy to humbly admit what we don't know, and where we lack data. Even if the health benefits of specific ingredients in infant formula are still up for debate, it's reasonable to spend some extra bucks on a fancier formula that fits your moral needs, your baby's palette, or just seems right for your little one. But it's *only* okay if that formula is safely manufactured, distributed, stored, and of course, nutritionally complete. Like you, pediatricians expect strict safety regulation of everything sold for infant consumption, just like any medication that we would prescribe. In the United States, this means only choosing a formula that meets all the requirements of the Infant Formula Act. Any option that comes through a third-party vendor—like those fancy, imported European formulas— bypasses the critical layers of consumer protections that this act was designed to create (and enforce!). Tampering prevention falls to the wayside, storage locations are unregulated, and the risk of bacterial contamination is significant—and something that outweighs any theoretical benefit of a plant-based protein or specific sugar substrate. Skipping internal regulation and Infant Formula Act protections also means that important recalls are missed or delayed, and recalls are quite common. The composition of these formulas isn't always the same as what the FDA recommends for babies in the United States, leading to certain vitamin and mineral deficiencies (hello iron, vitamin A, and copper!) that take effect before parents even realize they're lacking. Nothing is more important than your infant's safety, and if you're looking for a plant-based, European-style formula, make sure to stay local (yes, there are alternatives in the U.S.!) or talk to your pediatrician about other options. They may not have everything you want, but they're the best, safest way to give your baby everything they need.

An even more important caveat: When I say that considering a fancy, nonstandard formula is a reasonable option for most families, this does *NOT* include anything other than a commercial infant formula specifically engineered to meet the nutritional needs of babies. Reread that sentence, please. Any homemade, farm-bought, locally manufactured formula or milk product is a firm and final **NO**! I have to draw the line here, and I promise it's for your little one's safety. I've seen too many tragedies and watched too much suffering when extremely well-intentioned parents give milk products that are nutritionally incomplete, unsafely processed and stored, or both. I've seen infants fed with regular cow's milk, soy milk, almond milk, and goat's milk with devastating consequences. One six-month-old, whose parents were misinformed that unpasteurized goat's milk was appropriate for him, stayed admitted in the hospital for weeks with a life-threatening E. coli blood infection and liver damage from severe malnutrition. Another parent, after hearing the purported dangers of "chemically processed" commercial formula and the cow's milk protein it contains, switched her nine-month-old to almond milk with similarly devastating consequences. There's a lot we still don't know about infant feeding, and I humbly acknowledge that our understanding of optimal formula composition is just in its infancy. But there is absolutely no reason, ever, to explore these dangerous options.

The key to surviving baby fuss is to remember that it's okay to hate it. Almost all parents find themselves completely overwhelmed by their baby's cries at some (or many) points during those first few months. You're still a great, loving parent even if you acknowledge that inconsolable babies are caretaker torture machines. In most cases, your pediatrician will reassure you that your screaming baby is "safe," "healthy," and "normal." And while there may be nothing "wrong" with your baby, it's still okay to want to improve the situation. When the screaming ramps up, go ahead and try some of these safe and worthwhile interventions to help your baby calm down. Most important, take care of yourself through this truly challenging time. On my daughter's peak colicky days I used the money others spend on gas drops and fancy formulas to pay for a babysitter and a manicure. I tag teamed with my husband and as many other caretakers as possible. And if the screaming was just too much, I put her Safe to Sleep in her bassinet for thirty minutes, ignored the cries, and drowsily read a magazine and rested my aching shoulders. I did my best to practice what I preached, knowing that a happy and healthy parent is the most important ingredient in a developing baby's life.

THE BOTTOM LINE

5 out of 5 Pediatrician Parents Agree

- The majority of "fussy" babies are safe and healthy. But it can be miserable to deal with a screaming infant, and it's okay to be overwhelmed. Acknowledging the horrors of newborn fuss doesn't make you any less amazing a parent.

- Colic isn't dangerous, but it's still the worst. Strategic tag teaming, reducing light and noise in the home, and saving money for self-care and babysitters are the best strategies to handle this terrible rite of passage.

- Reflux is normal. If babies have a lot of pain or aren't growing, they might have GERD (gastroesophageal reflux disease).

- The best GERD treatment is giving smaller amounts of milk and keeping a baby upright after feeding. You should talk to a pediatrician before trying other strategies.

- Only babies with milk protein intolerance truly need special formulas. Fancy formulas aren't harmful, but they don't have any proven benefit.

- Any milk product or formula that isn't made specifically for infants' nutritional needs and manufactured and stored safely is an absolute **NO!**

PART TWO

3 to 6 Months

9

TAKE YOUR BEST SHOT

●●●●●●●●●●●●●●●●●●●●●●●●●●●●●●●●●●●●●●●

The Jury Is In on the Vaccine "Debate"

Many parents claim they aren't "anti-vaccine" but still talk about getting too many shots at once and "alternative" schedules. Worries may have changed—the fear of autism is out, concerns about too many "toxins" are in—but vaccine refusal is alive and growing (and only worsening in this pandemic, science-politicizing landscape). If I had a word limit, I'd summarize this topic with one simple sentence: Vaccines are the safest, most important intervention since clean drinking water, and all children deserve to be fully immunized according to the current schedule. Since I have the space, I'll talk about this at some length, mostly because: (1) there continues to be a criminal amount of compelling but false propaganda out there that is only growing in volume; and (2) this type of question is the rare example of when we, as doctors, do have a great, straightforward, 100% evidence-based answer where one option is actually the only right one.

Does this mean that I judge parents for asking critical questions? Of course not. There is so much worrisome misinformation out there, so it makes sense that parents remain skeptical. Early on in my training, I met Sarah, a sweet and precocious four-year-old girl who needed treatment for pneumonia. I remember my surprise when her mother told me she had refused all vaccinations. As a brand-new doctor, I could not reconcile this fact with her devotion to this smiling child. While Sarah and I colored and played together, her mother read excerpts from a variety of websites that carefully and convincingly put forth a false case against immunization. Even as a resident in pediatrics, I had trouble telling fact from fiction. But it was clear that Sarah's mother loved her more than anything. I promised to do my research and be prepared to answer not only her concerns, but also any and all questions that came up about vaccine safety. Over the years, I've seen thousands more patients, answered thousands of questions, and counseled thousands of families on the importance of vaccinations. I've done my research, and I am ready to give you the answers you need.

Start by taking a moment to ask yourself, why are you questioning vaccines? Each possible worry has been thoroughly debunked, and I'm here to provide a one-stop shop that explains the science in all its full, glorious detail.

The Greatest Vaccine Myths, Worries, Lies, and Assorted Misconceptions

"Vaccines Cause Autism"

If you're still fretting over any possible links to autism, made famous by the measles-mumps-rubella (MMR) vaccine and the now thoroughly disgraced and debunked claims of Andrew

Wakefield, one of medicine's greatest frauds, this is an easy one. Wakefield had multiple conflicts of interest, including financial gain from a competing vaccine maker, and created a falsified report to make it look like the MMR vaccine du jour was linked to autism. To put things in perspective, Wakefield's paper was a series of case reports (not even a study or trial) stating that twelve children who received the MMR vaccine were later diagnosed with autism. Let's compare that to a more recent analysis in 2014 that included data from over one million (yes, I mean million) children and found exactly zero relationship.

So why the increasing rates of autism in recent years? The best theories point toward factors such as parental age at conception (older people are having more kids these days), prenatal nutrition (our diets have changed significantly in the past decades), infection during pregnancy (some of which vaccines can prevent!), and prematurity (we're much better than we used to be at helping babies who are born early survive and thrive). In addition, pediatricians are much better at screening for autism now, and catching more cases than ever before. Even more important, the definition of autism has changed dramatically over the past decades, and children who would not have fit criteria even ten years ago are now placed on the spectrum.

"Kids Get Way Too Many Shots These Days"

Most of the parents I've seen who refuse or question vaccines are totally over the false link to autism. Instead, they ask questions like the following: Why are there so many more vaccines than there were when I was a kid? And couldn't all these shots hurt my baby and overwhelm their tiny immune system?

The simple answer is that there are more vaccines because science is awesome and we've been able to invent amazing lifesaving immunizations at a rapid rate. What's more, even though we now have vaccines for more diseases, we've been able to engineer them better, using fewer antigens, which is the part of the vaccine that mimics a virus or bacterium and triggers an immune response. So, contrary to popular belief, the immune system is not being exposed to some sort of crazy viral or bacterial orgiastic overload. I tell parents, accurately, that one visit for vaccines exposes their baby to fewer antigens than they would see if they touched a doorknob and then licked their hand. (And they will do this and far grimier things very frequently and from a very young age.) And since all vaccines have fewer antigens than the actual diseases, it is much more "overwhelming" for a baby's immune system to see a real-life virus or bacterium than to be vaccinated.

Okay, but isn't it stressful for a baby to have so many shots all at once? Many parents who do appreciate that vaccines are safe and important wonder about "alternative schedules," and feel that giving fewer vaccines at each visit is less traumatic for their little ones. But science disagrees. New studies show that giving all the vaccines at once is in fact less stressful because it's fewer separate instances of giving shots. And children who receive several vaccines at the same time don't have any more side effects or complications compared to children who get only one shot at a time.

More important, the current CDC schedule has been designed based on decades of research to create the safest and most protective vaccination plan for children. Babies have the weakest immune systems during their first year of life, as they begin to lose protection from antibodies that cross through the placenta. We vaccinate as soon as it's safe and effective to do so, protecting babies during a time when they are the most vulnerable.

"Natural Is Better"

The hardest myth to debunk is, as luck would have it, the most common reason for vaccine refusal. Nothing is more appealing than things that are "natural" these days, and even the best-informed parents are concerned that vaccinations are "chemical," "toxic," and "artificial." Some even ask why exposing their babies to the actual diseases wouldn't be a safer way to inoculate their little ones. Wouldn't it be better to build their immunity as Mother Nature intended—letting their body respond without giving a vaccine that has all these scary words like "antigens," "adjuvants," and "preservatives"?

Let's examine this at a few levels. First, all vaccine-preventable diseases are dangerous. Polio, tetanus, diphtheria—now essentially eliminated in our country due to uptake of their very effective vaccines—still claim the lives of tens of thousands of infants each year around the world due to a lack of access to timely vaccinations. And even diseases with a reputation for being "mild" often come at a serious price. Take chicken pox, caused by the varicella virus, which often resolves without complication and has the reputation for being little more than an itching inconvenience. Before the vaccine, seventy children died each year in the United States. That's more than have ever died from bacteria in an unwashed bottle, contaminated baby food, contaminated Romaine lettuce, or any outbreak you would take reasonable measures to prevent. And this is just one relatively "benign" illness. Measles, another "mild" childhood illness, caused hundreds of childhood deaths in the United States each year before a vaccine was invented. It's not just mortality, either. So-called mild viruses like varicella and measles can linger in kids' bodies, reemerging unpredictably years later to cause severe (think shingles) and even universally fatal (the nightmare of subacute sclerosing panencephalitis, a late complication of measles) devastation. It's clear that "natural" immunity is in fact much less safe, because the disease can kill or seriously harm, while the vaccine cannot.

There is also no reason at all to worry about the "toxins" and "chemicals" that the anti-vaccination misinformation machine has convinced parents pose a real threat to their baby's health. It's time to dig deeper into this fascination with "natural." There's a long-standing obsession with natural immunity, a fear of so-called toxins, and thinking that if something grows in nature it contains some sort of positive moral value. (Psychologists call this the "naturalistic fallacy.") Vaccines are a great example of the naturalistic fallacy in action. The anti-vaxx movement is centuries old. It's been cyclical, with people historically lining up to get their shots in times of epidemics (when the death toll made it hard to think of anything other than the need to prevent the horror around them, and with no social media to lead a politicized anti-vaccine propaganda campaign), then shying away due to fears of the exact same fantastical "toxins" when the fear of the disease itself abated.

Of course, "natural" is not always better. Babies used to die all the time from "natural" things like dysentery and even common colds before modern medicine. They still do. There is also no meaningful chemical difference between nature and medicine. Much of what we give as medicine is derived from plants with identical atomic structures, and much of what we find in nature is truly medicine with very real risks and benefits. The reality is that from a biochemical perspective, there is nothing different at all from your body seeing a virus or bacterium from the world as opposed to building immunity from the vaccine.

If that's too theoretical, metaphysical, psychological, or otherwise unconvincing, don't worry. I promise you that each component in every childhood vaccine is both necessary and completely safe. Predatory anti-vaccine groups have been devious in their ability to co-opt anxiety about the unknown, and the list of ingredients in vaccines have complex and (frankly) scary-sounding names that can terrify even the savviest parent. Anti-vaxx websites instruct parents to ask their pediatrician to review each item on the vaccine insert, promising a "gotcha" moment proving how dangerous they really are. But I review these ingredients in my daily practice when I counsel families, and I've never been "got."

To help demystify vaccines, I'll break down the components of vaccines so you can understand what those ingredients do.

A Is for Antigen!

Each vaccine contains an active ingredient, known as an "antigen," which is the part of the vaccine that allows the body to create an immune response. This part of the vaccine is either a whole virus or bacterium, a portion of a virus or bacterium, a chemical that the bacteria makes when it infects a person, or (excitingly and recently!) a molecule that tells your body to make one of those substances. The main concern I hear from parents about "antigens" is whether they can cause an actual infection. It's a good question, since they can contain actual parts of a bacterium or virus that causes serious illness. The short answer is no. Most childhood vaccines don't have any bacterial or viral particle that is even alive. There are five main ways that scientists can make an antigen that lets the body learn how to fight a disease without ever seeing the actual disease-causing organism.

Strategy 1: Use part of the virus/bacterium

The first way is what you'll see in vaccines that are called "subunit," "conjugate," "polysaccharide," or "recombinant." These are all words that describe the same concept: Scientists take just one component of the bacterium or virus—the part that the human body recognizes when it gets an infection and uses to make immune cells and memory—and isolate it from the rest of the virus or bacterium's disease-causing badness. There's no way your baby can get sick from these vaccines—like, ever— because there's no part of the vaccine that knows how to reproduce and infect their body. The only "downside" is that these types of vaccines don't produce as long-lasting an immune response, and often require more booster shots in adulthood.

Strategy 2: Inactivate the "toxin" bacteria make

The second method of making noninfective antigens is to create a "toxoid" vaccine. In this case, instead of using part of the disease-causing organism as an antigen, scientists inactivate the "toxin" that they make. Some very horrible diseases—famously tetanus and diphtheria, truly horrific illnesses that I thankfully have never seen—make a toxin when they infect you, and this is what your immune system fights when it gets sick. The inactivated toxin antigen, called a "toxoid," triggers the same immune response that a toxin would, but with none of the ability to hurt your baby's body. Again, there isn't any part of the bacterium or virus in these vaccines that can reproduce and get into cells, so it's not possible to get tetanus or diphtheria from it. It has literally never happened.

Strategy 3: Inactivate the whole virus or bacterium

The third method of making sure an antigen isn't active at all is . . . to inactivate it. This just means killing the bacterium or virus so that all the immune-producing parts are there, but it loses all its powers to infect you. How do we know this process works? Sadly, it's because of an extremely and famously horrible historical incident when this process went wrong. In 1955, hundreds of thousands of doses of the brand-new, lifesaving polio vaccines managed to leave the factory after a defective inactivation process. About forty thousand children contracted polio from the vaccine, two hundred were seriously ill, and ten died. It's an incredible tragedy that happened very, very early in our nation's vaccine manufacturing process. It's one of the many reasons the FDA is so strict about vaccine oversight, and there have been exactly zero cases of faulty inactivation since then.

Strategy 4: Weaken the virus or bacterium

Some vaccines do still contain very small amounts of technically "alive" virus in them. These are called "live-attenuated," and the only routine childhood vaccines that fall into this category are the MMR vaccine (measles, mumps, and rubella), varicella (chicken pox), and rotavirus. The best part of these vaccines is that the immunity your baby gets from them lasts a lot longer, so the majority of kids won't need any boosters at all when they grow up. The only downside is that for someone with an extremely weak immune system, they can "reactivate" and cause actual disease. Stressed? No need! The rotavirus vaccine is given orally to infants starting at two months. By then, any serious, extremely rare immune problem that makes this vaccine unsafe will be well-known to you and your doctor. In all my years seeing sick kids in the hospital, I've seen only one case where this vaccine was skipped. It was a child with severe combined immune deficiency (SCID), an extremely uncommon but very serious disease that is picked up either on the newborn screen (I told you, it's awesome!) or in the first weeks of life. Otherwise, every baby who gets the rotavirus vaccine does great. And while rotavirus might sound like a no-big-deal viral stomach bug, it's no joke. When babies do have rotavirus, even with modern medicine and all the IV fluids I can give them, they are sick for days or weeks, requiring long hospital stays. In other countries, viruses that cause diarrhea are actually the leading cause of death in infants. The MMR and varicella vaccines are similarly safe and are given for the first time at age six to twelve months to be extra sure that babies have an immune system that is ready to handle them.

Strategy 5: Let's get fancy with genetic codes (the virus's, not yours!)

The last, latest, maybe even greatest way to engineer an antigen is something you're already familiar with. Moderna's and Pfizer's covid vaccines are the most recent examples of how mRNA, an essential protein-coding molecule, can be used as an antigen. In this case, a vaccine contains a piece of mRNA that has been engineered to manufacture a specific protein. With covid vaccines, your body sees mRNA, your cells gobble it up, and then they use it to make the now-famous spike protein.

This spike protein signals a beautiful biochemical ballet in which your own human cells create covid immunity—without ever having to see the big, bad, covid-causing virus itself! This incredible dance is done in mere hours; the mRNA can't get into your DNA, into your RNA, or into anything dangerous before your cell's garbage disposal breaks it down and gets rid of it forever.

The other way that scientists take advantage of viral genetic codes is what you see in the other covid vaccines, and it's a similar concept. Instead of using mRNA to help your body prepare its immune system for a covid invasion, it uses DNA. The molecular properties of RNA and DNA are different, and in these cases we can't just rely on our cells to do the heavy lifting and take in the antigen in a carefully engineered soap bubble (which is more or less how mRNA is delivered). So to help us, scientists use something called a "viral vector." This doesn't have anything to do with the coronavirus itself. Instead, another common cold virus, most commonly "adenovirus," gets killed in a lab (RIP). Put some immunity-creating DNA in this deceased viral shell (which can't replicate or infect you, but still knows how to enter cells), and you get the same result as any other antigen: Your body sees something that belongs to the baddie you're trying to prevent, and learns how to fight it.

In conclusion, when vaccines are given according to the CDC schedule and to the right patients (which is all babies without an exceedingly rare contraindication), there is no chance that your baby can become sick with the disease they are working to prevent.

Amazingly, anti-vaccine groups spread misinformation not only that antigens are too strong, but also that they're somehow too weak. It's technically true that most infections cause a longer-lasting immunity than their vaccine counterparts. This is because most vaccines are engineered to have a lower "dose" of antigen compared to what your body would see in the wild. Some exceptions include HPV, pneumococcus, tetanus, haemophilus, influenza B, and the all-new, miraculous, pandemic-ending covid vaccines. But the reality is that this slightly shorter-lasting immunity is irrelevant for a few reasons. The first is that, as I mentioned, we have scheduled boosters that are given when you need a re-up! If you're in a high-risk field, like health care, you'll even get bloodwork that proves your immunity and get boosters more frequently if needed (raise your hand if you've had the MMR vaccine 5 times: 🙋🏻‍♀️). What's more, if we have good community uptake of a vaccine, we can essentially eradicate it, and it doesn't matter how long immunity lasts so long as we keep vaccinating before it has a chance to come back (unless a combination of amazing uptake and properties of disease transmission combine to let us completely eradicate a disease and stop vaccinating entirely, like with smallpox). Also, even if shorter-lasting immunity had an actual real-world impact, it's a clearly worthwhile trade-off. I said it once, and I'll say it again: Infections cause short- and long-term damage, while vaccines don't.

That's what you need to know about antigens. But what about the other items on that seemingly endless vaccine ingredient insert? These also fall into three different categories—adjuvants, stabilizers, and preservatives—and, like antigens, have been studied extensively. They are all completely safe to administer in the dosages contained in vaccines.

A Is Also for Adjuvant!

Adjuvants are substances that make the vaccine work better by causing a stronger immune response. This means that fewer doses of a vaccine are needed, and/or that we can give a smaller dose of the vaccine to your baby. In the United States, the three adjuvants used are aluminum salts, monophosphoryl lipid A, and squalene. Some anti-vaccine groups focus on aluminum, claiming that because it's a metal that makes it "toxic" and dangerous. Nope. The fun fact they ignore is that humans consume metals all the time. That phrase "vitamins and minerals," that your breakfast cereal uses to promote its health benefits? Those minerals are zinc, copper, iron, selenium, manganese, and other trace metals. Aluminum isn't a metal that your body needs in the same way, but it is absolutely found in normal foods and something we consume every day. Another fun fact: In the first six months of life, infants get more aluminum from breast milk or formula than they do from receiving all the routine vaccines combined.

Stabilize This

Vaccines also contain stabilizers, which are substances (sometimes just run-of-the-mill food products like gelatin) that help them last during production and transport. We think that stabilizers might be the component of vaccines that are responsible for extremely rare (as in a less than one in one million chance), serious, but treatable allergic reactions. They don't have any other side effects. Of course, that doesn't mean they haven't been the target of misinformation. When the amazing, cancer-preventing HPV vaccine came out, claims quickly emerged that its stabilizer, polysorbate 80, causes infertility. It doesn't. Polysorbate 80 is another crossover from the food industry and has been used in ice cream production for many years. A typical serving of ice cream has about 170,000 micrograms of polysorbate 80. Each dose of the HPV vaccine contains 50 micrograms. I'm not about to ban ice cream from my house, and I certainly won't be denying my daughter a cancer-preventing miracle over a little polysorbate 80.

Preservatives (a.k.a. the Case for Thimerosal)

The last type of ingredient is something you find in multidose vials, and this makes sense. Since we want these multiple-use containers to last longer, we need to add preservatives. Preservatives are extremely important and prevent contamination from other bacteria or even fungi. This was a big problem with the early vaccines, but thankfully, contaminated vaccines are a worry of the past. And like every other vaccine ingredient, each preservative we use has been extensively studied and proven to be completely safe.

The most famous preservative, thimerosal, became a topic of great controversy when Wakefield's acolytes proposed it was the ingredient linked to autism. Extensive research has proved this to be false, but even so, in 1997, the FDA decided to remove thimerosal from all childhood vaccines in the United States (with the exception of the multidose vial of the influenza vaccine) in an attempt to end the vaccine "debate" once and for all. By caving to anti-vaccine lobbies, scientists believed they could close the conversation. Instead, the anti-vaccine propaganda machine used this decision as ammunition to claim a victory, stating that thimerosal had been dangerous all along. And almost immediately, these anti-vaccine groups found new vaccine components to make erroneous and fear-based claims about. It was a bad political move, and thimerosal shouldn't make anyone think twice about the multidose flu shot.

In the end, there's only one right answer: Say yes to vaccines, give your baby all the vaccines, and give them on time. It's what I did for my daughter. I had zero hesitation or worry and left each visit relieved that she was safer from harm than when she had entered the office. And you should let yourself feel that way too. No late-night internet searching or play-group parental fearmongering needed; simply follow your pediatrician's advice without a second thought.

A Brief Note on the Covid Vaccine for Kids (and Why Getting Flu Shots for the Whole Family Is the Best Way to Kick Off Your Fall Festivities)

Oh, hello there. So glad you stuck around. I suppose you noticed a highly discussed, newsworthy, innovative, and essential vaccine casually slipping its way into our vaccine-ingredient discussion. But my guess is you'd like to hear a little bit more about these miraculous, pandemic-crushing vaccines as they specifically relate to your little one.

It's still surreal that I started to write this book before covid even existed, began finalizing this chapter before a vaccine was available, and am now finishing it when this lifesaving shot is *finally* available to kids. So let's talk about it.

By the time you're reading this, my prediction (and deepest wish) is that a covid vaccine will be approved and accessible to everyone six months old and up. And my other deepest wish is that parents around the globe will be lining up to protect their little ones with this amazing, lifesaving shot. Why am I so obsessed with the covid vaccines and why do I know that kids absolutely need to get their shots, just like adults? Because kids deserve protection from covid. Full stop.

There's way too much talk from pundits and politicians about if, how, and how much covid is a threat to kids. I understand wanting to keep worries in check during this pandemic. It's been a rough few years, to say the least. It's all too easy to get swept up in the endless anxiety. A little perspective makes sense, and reminding yourself that your kid's exposure to covid isn't the be-all and end-all of possible dangers is important.

The truth is that parenting is full of dangers, difficult choices, risk-benefit balances. Every decision we make balances the potential harms with the potential gains. With covid, this means staying on task and weighing the risks of covid to kids with the risks of the measures we take to prevent it.

What are the risks of covid transmission and infection? They don't need to be panic-inducing, but they are significant. Covid can affect children, and while the percentage of kids who get seriously sick from acute illness is much lower than adults, it's not zero. Remember, a small percentage of a big number is a big number! And of course, the harms of covid extend well beyond initial infection. Long covid is real and affects kids. Also, an overburdened health-care system will be unable to provide lifesaving care to all children who need it, not just kids with covid. Ongoing transmission creates more contagious variants, prolongs our pandemic, leads to school closures, quarantines, and otherwise delays the return to unrestricted play and education our children deserve.

These risks are worth preventing, and we know that covid vaccines prevent this—and how! Data from literally billions of people around the globe has shown that these vaccines are incredibly effective. We've seen jaw-dropping protection against infection and transmission, and an unprecedented ability to prevent serious disease and death. Safety data has been similarly impressive, continues to emerge, and any source claiming that the potential harms outweigh the benefits just hasn't done any actual research.

We can expect the same for kids. It's exactly what we've seen so far. Children tolerate the vaccine better, with fewer of those uncomfortable immediate side effects than we see in adults. Trials have been carefully designed to create and refine dosing, targeting the perfect balance that maximizes immune response and minimizes those aches and fevers that we see in the first days after vaccine administration. Reports of rare post-vaccine incidences that make splashy headlines—I'm looking at you, a very unhelpful, unscientific, unnuanced discussion of myocarditis—miss the mark. It's important to stay vigilant and to react quickly to any red flags. Adjusting schedules based on the risk of certain reactions (or choosing a different vaccine type; thank goodness there are so many options!) is something we expect. But it doesn't change the fact that the risks of vaccination are miniscule compared to the risks of covid. I've seen exactly zero cases of vaccine-induced myocarditis, and all reported cases have been treatable. I've seen countless cases, on the other hand, of covid-induced myocarditis, including older children who spent weeks on life-support and even a teenager who passed away.

The data is emerging, the science is evolving. I'm here for it. I've learned plenty of hard-earned lessons during this pandemic, and an important one has been just how little we've told parents about the limited evidence we have in pediatric medicine. It's a real issue (and a particular pitfall of "data-driven parenting") that leaves pediatricians using a lot of common sense, biology, and clinical expertise to decide how to help you keep your kids healthy. I'm truly excited to see so much research being done, so much focus on how to safely and effectively protect kids from covid. And the evidence we have is already so much more than we have for a huge number of treatments that we give to kids every day!

It's certainly infinitely more extensive and robust than the science we have behind any vitamin, supplement, pill, or medication that we use to treat covid (and a variety of other conditions) in kids. The anti-vaccine propaganda machine has made it all too easy to think we should deny children the protection they deserve from a highly studied vaccine, usually in order to sell whatever highly unstudied remedy they are trying to peddle instead. It's okay to just say "no," to refuse to get caught up in the unscientific hype. We are well past the pandemic point of no return, and covid is here to stay. The choice is between covid infection and vaccination, and the choice is crystal clear.

Same for the seasonal flu shot. The decision to get your yearly influenza protection—for your children, yourself, and all caretakers—can be a similarly un-agonizing one. We have decades more data to support just how safe this vaccine is for kids. Combine that with centuries of evidence that shows the devastating and deadly impact of flu in children (especially infants), and you'll quickly understand why I view this seasonal shot as just another crucial component of the routine childhood immunization series. No need to waste precious parental energy on an internal debate. Feel free to follow my lead, jump with joy when the flu shot becomes available every fall, and line the whole family up to get their dose of influenza protection.

THE BOTTOM LINE

5 out of 5 Pediatrician Parents Agree

- Vaccines are the safest and most important public health intervention since clean drinking water and citywide sanitation.

- They are given at times when it makes the most sense for little baby bodies to get them: before they are likely to see the disease and at a time when their body can mount a sufficient response, with boosters as needed to keep them protected.

  o All the components are safe.

  o There is no risk of overwhelming your baby's immune system.

  o There is nothing "better" about getting terrible and preventable diseases "naturally."

- Giving all the vaccines at once is less stressful for a child because there are fewer visits to the doctor's office for shots.

- The seasonal flu shot is just as important and safe as the other vaccines in the recommended childhood series—don't skip it!

- The covid vaccine is here for kids. I'm following the data closely and I continue to be impressed, excited, and recommend it for all children. They deserve to be protected from vaccine-preventable disease!

10

TO SLEEP TRAIN, PERCHANCE TO DREAM

•••

Why It's Completely Okay
(but Still Not Mandatory)
to Let Your Baby Cry at Night

No parenting book is complete without a chapter on "sleep training," grinding through the nuts and bolts of teaching an infant how to sleep through the night. But instead of comparing side-by-side sleep training techniques, touting a favorite, or even creating a new one, this chapter will dive deep into much more fundamental concerns. First, I'll answer the most basic, and most ignored, parental question: Should you sleep train your baby? I'll explain why in most situations the answer is yes, but not for the reasons you've been told. While pediatricians, bloggers, and guidebooks all obsess over infant sleep, focusing on a parent's sleep is the most important part of raising a happy and healthy baby. I'm here to prove that prioritizing your own rest is reason enough for you to embrace sleep training. I'll also show you why sleep training techniques are more alike than they are different, and that the right approach for your baby is simply the one that you'll feel comfortable following.

Before explaining why sleep training is the right choice for most parents, and what benefits it does and does not provide, let's debunk the two biggest myths.

Myth #1: Letting a Baby Cry at Night Is Child Abuse

Of course it's not. This lie was promoted—and is still perpetuated—by those ascribing to a philosophy known as "attachment parenting," a method popularized in the 1980s by Dr. William Sears. Ah, that crazy time called the eighties, when shoulder-padded, pantsuit-clad women entered the workforce in increasing numbers. At the same time, Dr. Richard Ferber released his famous sleep training guide, *Solve Your Child's Sleep Problems*, a book so popular that any technique that approximates his methods is still referred to as "Ferberizing." And as you may remember from Chapter 7, the 1980s saw a peak in exclusive formula feeding. The result was a reality where mothers were physically holding their babies less than ever. This increased distance between mother and baby was the key driver behind the success of the "attachment parenting" movement. Popularized by Dr. Sears, this philosophy states that if parents constantly maintain physical contact with their babies—and consistently respond to their cues and cries—their infants will form healthy attachments and have optimal emotional well-being.

While the idea of restoring snuggle time seems like a great idea, "attachment parenting" has deep flaws. Its origins remain problematic, with Dr. Sears basing his approach on less-than-scientific studies on the parenting habits of native cultures in Bali and Zambia. He used these anthropological observations to justify his approach, glorifying the "natural" parents he observed without caring to learn much about their cultures. His philosophy is also heavily founded in a particular Christian model of traditional female domesticity. Even many modern organizations that preach variations on attachment parenting remain steeped in religious identity and the promotion of a woman's primary role as a homemaker.

Practicing attachment parenting also poses real logistical challenges, demanding that parents (especially mothers) can always be physically touching their babies. This ignores the reality of life for most new parents, assuming that their work allows them to spend months and months at home, that they don't have lives of their own that might take them away from their little one, and that there's a "village" of caretakers able to tag in when parents need even a few hours of me time.

Attachment parenting is expectedly pro-bed-sharing, as this allows for both maximizing physical touch and constant response to an infant's cries. Unfortunately, but unsurprisingly, attachment parenting advocates have found that equating sleep training with child abandonment is an excellent way to convert parents to their approach—and to monetize their "free advice" by selling countless products to help parents constantly cuddle their little ones. The "scientific" harms that attachment parents use to support this claim originated from an outrageously irrelevant study. It showed that infants in orphanages, where they were largely ignored, had minimal interaction and nurturing, and were allowed to cry for hours on end, later developed severe behavioral and emotional problems. It's a truly tragic paper to read, but anyone who thinks this somehow proves that sleep training is akin to this type of neglect—as I've seen countless parents do in forums across the internet, and even written in official parenting guides—clearly hasn't read it (or have any basic understanding of the scientific method).

The Attachment Parenting International group has modernized a bit, and its website has now replaced the Romanian orphanage study with a new study from 2011. This one, led by University of Texas's Dr. Wendy Middlemiss, showed higher cortisol (a stress hormone) levels in babies whose parents did strict "cry it out" sleep training (which is a very specific, extreme technique). It's an important finding but misses so much of the nuance of this discussion. For starters, most parents can't tolerate this black-and-white "cry it out" approach. We also don't know if this elevated cortisol is a bad thing (people produce higher levels in stressful situations, but that doesn't mean that there is any long-term damage). Maybe it's even an important part of helping babies build distress tolerance, which is a scientifically plausible—if still theoretical—benefit to sleep training.

The studies pediatricians cite, on the other hand, suggest that a gradual sleep training approach is indeed safe. For example, a landmark 2012 Australian study found no differences in baby's behavior, development, stress regulation, bonding to parents, and even maternal mental health in babies whose parents were taught a gradual sleep training technique. The only actual randomized trial studying sleep training was done by Dr. Lisa A. Adams in 1989 and demonstrated that gradual sleep training not only worked but also helped marriages (which came as a surprise to exactly zero parents). There's simply no evidence that a modified gradual approach to sleep training (like the one popularized by Dr. Richard Ferber) has any harmful effects.

Another fun fact: Sleep training doesn't mean abandoning attachment-promoting techniques altogether. There are plenty of other ways to engage in attachment-style parenting for parents who dig that philosophy but just need to get a little more sleep. Baby wearing, indulging daytime screams, and general love and affection are all still on the table. Just ask my daughter, whose strict sleep training didn't interfere in the least with my giving her almost hourly snuggles, kisses, hugs, hair brushing, and songs of praise and love that are finally starting to embarrass her. The evidence is clear: Parents who sleep train can be as loving as those who don't.

Myth #2: Sleep Training Is Mandatory for Raising a Strong, Resilient Baby

Nope. While sleep training is safe, and doesn't deprive a baby of any affection, parents need to understand that it isn't magic. I've counseled countless parents who put tremendous pressure on themselves to start sleep training at the exact-right time, using the exact-right system, and do it in the exact-right way. They've heard that perfect adherence to sleep training is a scientific necessity that will create worry-free infants, providing a real psychological and emotional benefit to their little one. I remember one mom who came to her daughter's one-month-checkup with three sleep training books in hand, anxious to find out which was the best way to get her baby on a strict sleep schedule as soon as possible. Before diving into a side-by-side guide comparison, I asked if there was any particular reason that she was so eager to start her baby's bedtime routine. She paused, answering that she hadn't really thought about it. She assumed that it was somehow important for her daughter's health to learn how to sleep through the night at an early age, since this is what friends, family, and even her night-nurse had told her.

The idea that sleep training is good for a baby's well-being is based on concepts from the world of clinical and behavioral psychology. Sexy stuff, I know, but it really is important to have a handle on this background, because it informs how sleep training methods continue to win over parents. Child and behavioral psychologists have posited that sleep training could help build distress tolerance—a psychological term that simply means a person's ability to manage stressors—which is now thought to be a key part of why some people have fewer mental health issues than others. Our understanding of distress tolerance has led to the creation of a whole field of therapy called resilience training—a broad term encompassing a variety of techniques that help people learn how to improve their own distress tolerance. There's no actual, direct link to sleep training. Rather, the hypothesis is that through teaching a baby to learn to self-soothe from an early age, sleep training provides a foundation in distress tolerance and could even serve as a booster shot of resilience training.

But we don't have any evidence that sleep trained babies have more resilience later in life, and there are other ways to raise a strong, well-adjusted baby. For now, at least, the science isn't there, and building resilience isn't a good enough reason to say "yes" to sleep training.

But sleep training sells. In one corner, attachment advocates prey on your parental guilt, claiming that sleep training is terrible for a baby's emotional well-being. The rebuttal—that sleep training isn't just safe, but it's somehow crucial to raising a happy and healthy baby—is an effective way to keep parents from jumping off the sleep training bandwagon. None of this means sleep training isn't important to discuss—or even promote. In fact, I strongly encourage embracing sleep training to almost every family that I counsel on the topic. Why? Because though sleep training isn't required to raise an emotionally adjusted child, the single proven, scientific benefit of sleep training is that it gives parents more quality sleep.

Parents, like all humans, need good, uninterrupted sleep to stay alert during the day. An attachment parent may be constantly cuddling their baby, or even quickly responding to their cries both day and night. But the well-rested parent is often more engaged during play, stays awake and interactive during snuggles, sings louder, dances with more vigor, and otherwise has enough energy to do all the incredibly important daytime activities that babies need to bond, grow, and thrive. In addition, sleep helps anxiety, and parental anxiety is a known factor for emotional distress in babies (and even can lead to long-term health consequences in older children). And sleep deprivation, as mentioned in Chapter 6, is its own risk factor for SIDS. In the end, it's clear that your rest as a parent is crucial to your baby's health.

How to Choose a Sleep Training Technique

Convinced that sleep training is right for you? Great! Now it's time to stay chill as you are bombarded with hundreds of supposedly unique sleep training methodologies. It's overwhelming. Guidebooks, blog posts, pricey sleep consultants, and even some pediatricians all claim that there's one single, best approach that will teach any baby how to sleep through the night. But the truth is that the majority of these techniques are much more alike than they are different. These similarities mean that any sleep training recipe that has a few basic ingredients is as good as any other. It's why the "best" sleep training system for you is simply the one you'll feel comfortable following.

To truly understand the components of effective sleep training, you'll need another very brief primer in behavioral psychology. You might remember from Psych 101—at least vaguely—how behavior can be shaped through strict routines. It's something we learned from animals, starting with classical conditioning and Pavlov's famous dogs, to operant conditioning and Skinner's decidedly less-famous pigeons. The basic premise is that by promoting associations, reinforcing certain behaviors, and ignoring undesired ones, we can dramatically and effectively shape the actions of almost any animal. Including humans.

After learning how easily they could influence dogs and pigeons, behavioral psychologists turned to people. This meant babies, too, and it's these same behavioral psychologists who originated the idea of sleep training altogether. One of the earliest to do so was Dr. James Watson, whose teachings were exceedingly popular as early as the 1890s. Watson and others ascribed to a very strict (and very incorrect) theory that every aspect of a child's development is based on learned behaviors. To them, this meant that it was in fact necessary for infants to cry overnight, and that ignoring this crying was the only way a baby could ever learn how to sleep through the night. This is where the "cry it out" philosophy originated, with Dr. Emmett Holt's 1894 book outlining how tolerating unlimited crying (without any amount of comforting) was the only way to go. Today's "cry it out" or pure-extinction method advocates espouse a virtually unchanged approach: simply place a calm but still awake baby in their crib, close the door, and return only in the morning. Crying can last for hours and hours, but in just a few days, it is in fact true that your baby is going to sleep like an angel for the whole night.

The next decades saw an explosion of parenting guides, books, and an entire new class of "parenting experts," many of whom—most famously Dr. Spock—fought back against strict infant scheduling, including "cry it out." The pendulum swung back and forth until 1985, when that definitive sleep training authority, Dr. Richard Ferber, published his first edition of *Solve Your Child's Sleep Problems*. Ferber echoed some earlier themes of sleep-behavior modification, stressing the importance of consistent bedtime rituals (a fixed routine to promote associations), but stopped short of pure extinction and spared parents endless overnight baby screams. Ferberized baby screams, rather, are still present, but do have an endpoint. At bedtime, parents place their calm but awake baby in their crib and then leave the room. But after a certain amount of screaming (for example, three minutes), the parent comes back into the room to comfort the baby without picking them up. After the first return, each subsequent calming-session comes a little later—five minutes, then ten minutes, then twelve minutes, and so on. At a certain point, all babies give up and fall asleep.

Since Ferber, hundreds of other techniques have emerged, most of which are little more than modified "Ferberization." This includes "camping out," which lets parents stay in the room, lying down next to their baby's crib, soothing them with patting or stroking, then leaving only when they fall asleep. It's all variations on a theme, and still works toward the goal of helping a baby learn that they can in fact fall asleep (and stay asleep) all on their own. Any effective sleep training approach has the same basic components that make behavioral conditioning successful: creating fixed routines to help them form associations between bedtime and sleep, reinforcing desired behaviors (like actually saying, "Good morning, baby! I'm so proud of you for sleeping by yourself!"), ignoring or minimizing response to undesired behaviors (like crying when they're alone in their crib), and creating a safe environment for their little brains to figure this all out.

So which sleep training technique is the best? The Ferber method and its modern variations hold the title for me. Some sleep trainers still swear by cry it out, but this has become increasingly less popular as more gradual techniques have proven to be just as effective and usually less miserable for parents. I have met few parents who can power through the hours of strict "cry it out" screaming, while the gradual, Ferber-esque techniques are far less emotionally draining—and work just as well. And a Ferberizing parent, on average, gets more sleep themselves than the "cry it out" parent who has been up for as many as five hours in a row. Any chosen method only works when the steps are implemented consistently, meaning whichever you feel you'll be able to follow is the right choice for you. It's key to stick to the plan, but your decision is just for a moment in time. If follow-through just isn't happening (I get it! It's hard!), stop, regroup, and modify your approach. There's no sense in powering through ineffective sleep training. When you do it, make it count.

Of course, there are a few caveats when considering which sleep training method is right for you. For example, while the pea-sized newborn stomach grows quickly the first few months, many babies remain truly hungry for an overnight feed until they are four months old. This means that some of the most popular systems—some of which even promise an uninterrupted twelve hours of sleep by a baby's three-month birthday—face an uphill battle. Waiting to start sleep training in earnest—around three months is a good time to dive in—makes a lot more sense.

This doesn't mean that you can't lay the groundwork early on. In my first depressed, anxious, exhausted postpartum months, I remember asking my supervising doctors constantly when I should start sleep training, my scientific question masking a desperate plea for permission to try something, anything that would get me more sleep. Yes, true sleep training was unlikely to succeed until the three- to four-month mark, they confirmed, but I was empowered to start practicing our consistent bedtime routine as early as I wanted. It really laid the groundwork, and helped me gain some control of bedtime from the screaming chaos that once sent me into fits of panic. By two months, we had all sunk into the comfort of a nightly feed, two books in the rocking chair, diaper change, swaddle, bedtime song (we still sing the exact same one every night over four years later), sound machine, lights off, then back to sleep. We opted out of certain popular bedtime routine ingredients like bathtime (a very unsoothing event for my bath-phobic little one) and blackout curtains (which I knew I'd be too lazy to tote around on trips in the future when she would likely become accustomed to sleeping with them). She often cried immediately, and we picked her up within minutes, saving our scream-tolerance for when sleep training was officially in process about six weeks later. Yet it was something we could do as a family, giving me an ounce of control over the evening's madness, and bringing hope as we prepared for more sleep-filled nights that were soon to come.

New parents, I see you. I was you, a brand-new mother beyond exhausted, conflicted, confused, and uniquely susceptible to bad information. It's okay to ignore it all. Instead, you can opt into sleep training—and choose whatever approach matches your style—without an ounce of unnecessary stress.

THE BOTTOM LINE

5 out of 5 Pediatrician Parents Agree

- Sleep training is not child abuse.

- Sleep training doesn't have any proven psychological, emotional, or resilience-building benefits.

- Sleep training is still worthwhile—for almost every modern parent, it's a necessary ingredient to restoring parental sleep, which is reason enough to love it. Well-rested parents are happier and healthier and raise happier and healthier babies.

- Babies usually wake up overnight to eat until they are at least three months old, so you should wait to start sleep training until then. Starting a bedtime routine before that is a good option to lay the groundwork and regain a sense of calm, control, and hope for sleep-filled nights to come.

- Any sleep training system that you can follow through with is the right one for you. The majority of parents prefer a gradual approach, so it likely makes sense to choose something Ferber-adjacent to start.

11

THE TRUTH ABOUT PACIFIERS

• •

Why Your Baby's Binky Addiction Is Very Real (but Nothing to Worry About)

It's painful to admit, but there was a time when I judged parents whose toddlers were still using pacifiers. My logic was simplistic: Pacifiers are for babies! The American Academy of Pediatrics recommends stopping pacifier use by age two, and I was taught to counsel parents to start the weaning process (or at least plan for it) at their one-year checkup. Other sources—like the ear, nose, and throat doctors I worked with, or the American Academy of Family Physicians—enforced a strict ban by age one, and on rotations with specialists I told parents to start their wean as early as six months old.

Of course, the truth is that the pacifier debate is as nuanced as any other. Isn't it wild that despite all the advances in pediatric medicine, the controversies surrounding topics as basic as pacifier use are as heated as ever? Never fear, I'm here to tackle all your burning binky questions.

Let's start by reviewing all the good we know pacifiers can do (besides the obvious baby-soothing role they play in any exhausted new parent's life). There's one main, important, studied benefit to giving binkies to tiny babies: lower chances of SIDS. In 2005, the American Academy of Pediatrics looked at nine of the decade's best studies. They found that these studies, which compared babies who died of SIDS with healthy counterparts, all showed that fewer babies in the SIDS group were put to bed that night with a pacifier in their mouth. The famous New Zealand study we talked about in Chapter 6, which teased apart the different SIDS risk factors, even found that one of the strongest protective factors was in fact pacifier use. It's not definitive, but it's a promising connection. And it makes sense with what we understand about SIDS, which is known to be related to how babies' brains coordinate breathing. Sucking on a pacifier makes babies sleep less deeply, increasing their response to things that can go wrong (like forgetting to breathe). They also help babies breathe through their mouths if their noses get blocked and change the position of their tongues so they are less likely to block their airways. Whatever the reason, the data is compelling, and something that might have some role in preventing SIDS is hard to ignore.

So why not let your child use a pacifier for as long as they want, especially if it might play some role in preventing SIDS? There are a few potential harms that have ignited the binky controversy in pediatricians' offices and on parenting message boards alike. The first is teeth, with many worried that extended pacifier use will cause serious damage to those tiny, adorable pearly whites. But after decades of anecdotal evidence that binky addictions cause cavities and crooked teeth, recent studies have put this common misconception to the test. Today's pediatric dentists agree that pacifier use only leads to tooth decay when parents give babies binkies sweetened with sugar or juice. As for unsweetened plastic? The latest data has consistently shown that sugar-free pacifiers only lead to cavities and gum disease when used for a *very long* time. Most studies don't see any significant risk until age three years, and many not until age five! Furthermore, it seems that any changes in tooth alignment from early pacifier use are likely reversible if weaning happens before permanent teeth come in—usually around kindergarten.

What's more, most children whose pacifiers are taken away quickly replace this habit with another, swiftly learning to suck thumbs, fingers, or chew on whatever is in sight. In fact, most dentists prefer pacifiers because it's easier for a parent to control when and how much a baby chews on a pacifier than a finger, and much easier to wean a binky addiction than a thumb-sucking habit. And replacing plastic with skin opens a whole new world of infection and blisters. While you might be thinking that this is common and no big deal—which often is true—there are cases where it causes real problems. Just ask Jayden, a three-year-old boy who I treated in the hospital with IV medication for a particularly nasty, painful infection called herpetic whitlow that he received courtesy of unstoppable thumb-sucking. The true baby teeth experts routinely give pacifiers to their own children for these exact reasons.

Another oft-cited risk of early pacifier use is an association with ear infections. The American Academy of Family Physicians continues to cite this risk as the main reason for promoting a pacifier wean at six months old, and pediatric ear, nose, and throat doctors frequently discourage pacifier use altogether. Some studies do, in fact, suggest that babies who use pacifiers have more ear infections than those who don't, but the underlying data is shaky. For example, in 1995, Finnish researchers divided around nine hundred babies in day care centers into two groups. They counseled parents in one group that pacifiers could be harmful and didn't tell the other group anything. Later, they found that the families who were counseled on pacifier risks were less likely to enforce an outright pacifier ban—but the parents in this "counseled" group didn't give pacifiers as frequently. They also saw that this group of babies was a little less likely to get ear infections than the group that had received no counseling. Their conclusion: using pacifiers more frequently leads to ear infections.

Confused? Me too. The study design makes it impossible to draw any real conclusions. Others are similarly weak. Some simply look at a group of babies and see how many used pacifiers and how many had ear infections, concluding that pacifier use and ear infections are related. But these observational studies make it difficult to draw conclusions about causation, as there are far too many other factors that could be contributing. Pacifier use is related to breastfeeding, and breastfeeding is related to ear infections, and all of these are related to socioeconomic status. So while data suggests there *may* be a relationship, there's not enough evidence yet to use the fear of ear infections as justification for binky bans.

Even if good data existed, it's important, as always, to think about how much this risk should be a deterrent against pacifier use. It's another great example of where numbers don't matter if the risks and benefits are nowhere near close to being equally important. Did the possibility of my having an extra ear infection outweigh the benefits of a crucial soothing device that might even protect against SIDS? No way.

Okay, dental problems and ear infections aren't good enough reasons for a full pacifier ban starting on your baby's first birthday. What else have the medical and parenting worlds thrown at you to make what seems like a relatively easy decision—give a baby their binky—turn into an agonizing exercise in new-parent guilt? The latest is all about breastfeeding.

A recent incarnation of "breast is best" evangelism comes in the form of the Baby-Friendly Hospital Initiative. It's a well-intentioned movement that strives to help hospitals—who still frequently separate babies from their parents, push formula willy-nilly into newborn mouths, and otherwise forget how to nurture the parent-infant bond—make breastfeeding support a priority. There are some interventions that make a lot of sense: The initiative helps keep babies with their parents for the first few hours after birth, provides universal lactation support, and lets babies stay in the same room as their parents for as much as possible while they are in the hospital. But some of the rules are essentially nonsense, none more so than the complete pacifier ban for all babies in the newborn nursery.

In a misguided attempt to help support breastfeeding, some pediatricians and lactation consultants now forbid pacifiers for all babies in the first weeks after birth. This practice is based on the assumption that early binky use makes it more difficult for babies to learn how to latch, and that parents are less likely to understand and respond to hunger cues appropriately if placing a pacifier in a crying mouth is an available option. But there is limited science, and while studies show that babies who use pacifiers starting in the first weeks of life end up weaning from breastfeeding earlier than those who don't, it's a correlation without a clear explanation.

One Quebec study had a similar design to that convoluted ear infection study, dividing infants into a group that was counseled not to use pacifiers to calm their (seemingly hungry) babies and a group with no counseling. The result was that the counseling decreased pacifier use, but that this decreased pacifier use didn't have any impact on breastfeeding rates or duration. Other research does show that using binkies is related to decreased breastfeeding, but these studies are all observational. To their credit, their authors draw very fair conclusions: They propose that frequent pacifier use doesn't necessarily cause breastfeeding problems, but more likely is an indicator that breastfeeding struggles are happening for some other reason (leading parents to place a pacifier in a baby's mouth rather than put them at the breast).

My daughter was born at the same hospital I worked in, which was already an officially designated Baby-Friendly hospital. Even before she was born, I was obsessively worried about SIDS, and I was on board with anything that might be able to prevent it. So despite my breastfeeding difficulties—spurred by prematurity, trouble latching, jaundice, and low blood sugars necessitating formula supplementation—I wasn't deterred from placing a contraband binky into her tiny mouth. I had made a calculated risk vs. benefit assessment for me and my daughter, and all signs pointed to plastic pacification. But SIDS risk aside, it's clear that the binky-breastfeeding connection is overblown.

As we reviewed in Chapter 7, optimizing breastfeeding requires being thoughtful about how pacifiers are used in the first few weeks, but there's no need to ban them altogether.

While breastfeeding interference, ear infections, and dental damage aren't reason enough to say no to plastic pacification, there is one major downside to enabling your baby's binky habit: quitting. Pacifiers work, and they work incredibly well. So well that after a few months of use, brains can develop a strong attachment and even verified addiction. It's what happened to my daughter. It's crazy to think that there was ever a time where I was the one pushing the pacifier on her as she lay in her bassinet, bundled for a night of the safest sleep I could conjure. By a few months of age, she refused to nap without one. When her binky dropped out of my hand and down a gutter on our way to day care, I thought we'd try the day without it. The result was a morning in which my daughter crawled around her class, plucking pacifiers out of her friends' mouths and placing them into her own (In a pre-pandemic world, this was mostly hilarious and at worst slightly embarrassing). I went to the pharmacy, purchased a replacement, and brought it to her before naptime. I should have never underestimated the power of the pacifier.

At my daughter's eighteen-month well-child visit, I hid her pacifier in my purse. I had nodded along to her pediatrician at the one-year checkup, as she counseled on the need to start weaning. I smiled and said I was planning on starting that month (I wasn't). It was an unnecessary lie, and my pediatrician would have understood. But the internet shame-machine had gotten to me, and I couldn't risk the chance that my honesty would be met with anything other than unconditional support. We had just made a big move to a new state, started a new childcare routine, were dealing with toddler sleep regression, and both her father and I were acclimating to new jobs. Removing the piece of plastic that she relied on to sleep, travel, or stop screaming in the middle of a supermarket was something I simply didn't have the bandwidth to do.

Shortly after my daughter's second birthday, my husband and I decided it was time to take the plunge. And while weaning wasn't a walk in the park, it was far less traumatic than I had feared. We started by transitioning pacifier use to strictly at bed and naptime only, with her nanny and day care teachers helping to keep this consistent rule. The tantrums were intense but short-lived. Within days, she knew that binkies were for bedtime and stopped asking at other times. A month later, after needless obsessing over the seemingly inevitable nightmare of removing her nighttime pacifier, we took the final leap. We thoroughly prepared her for days in advance— "now that you're a big kid, we need to give your pacifiers to the other babies to use, and you'll be able to sleep on your own and be just as safe as always"— then one night simply put her to bed empty-mouthed. Prepared for endless screams, I was met with whines and whimpers that quickly subsided into slumber. We repeated our pep talk for a few more nights until the memory of her precious piece of plastic seemed to have completely vanished. It wasn't a fluke; since then, I've counseled countless parents on how to use these sorts of techniques to kick their babies' binky habits, with similar success.

THE BOTTOM LINE

5 out of 5 Pediatrician Parents Agree

- Pacifier use is linked to reduced rates of SIDS, and while the relationship isn't definitively cause-and-effect, it is strong enough, and important enough, to count as a "pro" in the binky debate.

- Pacifiers don't cause cavities unless they are dipped in sweetener. They also don't cause any permanent dental problems unless they're used for a long time, at least past the third birthday.

- There's no firm rule on when pacifiers absolutely need to be weaned, but aiming to quit by around age three will prevent almost all possible long-term effects.

- Pacifier use early on is related to breastfeeding problems, but this is a correlation and not enough reason to ban newborn binkies.

- Worries over ear infections aren't reason enough to ban pacifiers.

- Pacifiers pacify. The biggest "pro" in the paci debate is that they are extremely effective at soothing screaming babies.

- Pacifiers are indeed addictive, and weaning is challenging— but you'll be able to use a few simple techniques to kick your toddler's binky habit with minimal stress.

- It's simply okay to embrace pacifier use, and your little one's inevitable addiction is completely pediatrician and mom approved (for at least a few years).

12

BUY THE BOOK

• •

Building Your Baby's Library and Promoting an Early Love of Reading

Pediatricians love nothing more than handing a newborn one of their very first board books at their first office checkup. I have yet to meet a pediatrician whose office isn't filled with enough Dr. Seuss and Eric Carle to stock a library. Yet many parents may wonder why we medical doctors care so much about reading to a child who can barely keep their eyes open. There is a surprising amount of science on why babies should get to know their local library earlier than you might think. The good news: raising a book lover is even easier than it looks. Let's dive into the important pediatric topic of "early literacy," learning just how fun and simple it can be to turn your tiny newborn into a certified bibliophile.

The infant checkup visits that I performed during my residency training were as much about parenting as they were about medicine. After listening to a baby's heart and before giving a round of vaccines, I sat with parents and provided counseling. While I learned later as an exhausted and overwhelmed parent that some advice was either unrealistic or out of touch, the advice I gave about early reading was actually the same as what I followed when my daughter was born.

I recall one set of parents who couldn't help but roll their eyes when I asked how many books were at home and how often someone read to their baby. Their faces seemed to say, "Is this a doctor's visit or a preschool interview?" A one-month-old can't even follow someone's voice consistently. How can reading be essential medicine?

Early literacy is in fact important, but not for the reasons you've probably been told. No need to make literacy a competitive sport: Early reading won't turn your infant into a baby genius who can finish Proust before preschool. Instead, promoting an early love of books is simply a fun, easy way to engage in normal growth and development. The complex process of reading—including holding (or even chewing) a book, turning a page, following a story, repeating sounds, bringing attention to objects on a page, and following a narrative—enhances fine motor, social, and problem-solving skills.

There's already robust scientific literature (no pun intended) that demonstrates the ways in which exposing even the tiniest of infants to books and reading has real benefits. For example, in 2001, researchers at New York University randomized 122 children into two groups and provided half of them with intensive early literacy promotion through the Reach Out and Read program. They found not only that the program was effective in increasing how much parents read to their children at home, but they also found that there was a direct relationship between how much families read together and a child's ability to understand and express language. Other nonprofit programs, like Get Ready to Read!, Raising Readers, First Book, and even Dolly Parton's Imagination Library, all have similar missions and cite similar success stories. Socioeconomic status certainly plays a big factor in school readiness, but studies continually show that even for kids from the same socioeconomic background, with the same access to educational resources and opportunities, early reading really does improve language development. For example, researchers at the State University of New York looked at the homes of more than two hundred children and found that even controlling for socioeconomic status, the degree to which their families promoted reading was directly related to their language test scores, school readiness assessment, and even an ongoing interest in reading.

Early literacy doesn't just improve language acquisition (including vocabulary, grammar, storytelling, and fluency), but also translates into additional and long-lasting benefits. In another study, psychologists from the University of California, Berkeley and the University of Toronto teamed together to follow a group of fifty-six children from first grade through high school. They found that exposure to printed literature at home not only predicted reading scores in the first grade, but was able to predict scores through the eleventh grade—even when other measures of a child's reading comprehension were removed from the equation.

I'm not here to simply herald data; now that I've convinced you of the importance of helping your baby become an early reader, let's learn how to achieve this fun and easy milestone. The key to making early literacy a joy and not a chore is remembering that, just like any other parenting task, you can only control what you can control. And the most important thing that you can control is the book-loving environment that you create. Whether it's with newly purchased books, registry gifts, hand-me-downs, or through free books-for-kids programs like the nonprofits mentioned above, it's usually feasible and affordable to have a mini children's library ready to go by the time your little one arrives home.

Some creative storage, interior design, and decidedly unsubtle arrangement of books around the spaces your baby will explore is the next important step. Seasoned pediatrician parents generally embrace mess, and are especially accepting of an unkempt living space if it means that books are scattered across all sorts of corners, surfaces, and in easily accessible bins and boxes low to the floor. I was one of many pediatrician parents who took advantage of captive car commuting as a literacy-promoting experience. Yes, tablets sometimes won out (we'll talk about this in full, permissive detail in Chapter 13), but most days my daughter spent the drive to day care happily perusing whatever board books I had left next to her car seat. Throw a couple of books in the bottom of your stroller, in your diaper bag, on play mats, rugs, and couches, and your baby will be a certified early reader in no time.

Another thing you can control?—which books you choose to keep in your house. The best book for a baby is the book that their caretakers enjoy reading themselves. For infant literature, the bar is relatively low, and anything with some combination of attractive illustrations, pleasant rhyme, and a positive message became my personal favorite (until the hundredth time reading it, at which point the next good-enough book took its place).

It's also crucial to remember just how much of a comprehensive, immersive sensory exploration reading is for infants. This is why books with different textures, shapes, pop-ups, and features are all so much fun to discover. It's also why even more traditional book-like books will be used by your baby in the exact same way. Expect your infant to lick, chew, rip, crumple, and otherwise destroy any book they find. It's something to not only accept, but to celebrate. If you have a particularly valuable edition, a book with a personal inscription, or have otherwise attached sentimental value to one of your baby's books, place it away for later and focus on experimenting with replaceable reading for at least that first year of your little one's life.

If you're thinking, that's a lot that I can do to promote an early love of books, you're correct. So what on earth could be out of your control, and how could it be possible that your baby might not immediately fall in love with the literature you provide? While most babies will happily explore their libraries for longer than their caretakers will maintain interest, don't forget that babies are babies. All little ones are different, and every infant has their own mysterious likes, thoughts, whims, wishes, and feelings that dictate when, where, how much, and for how long a book will hold their attention. Don't force it. As we'll dive into in Chapter 17, promoting healthy habits means providing good choices, modeling good behavior, and practicing what you preach. Your own love of reading, your joint exploration of books, the pro-literacy environment that you have created are all your baby needs to reap the full benefits of early literacy—on their time and on their terms. Turning reading into a battle is at best unhelpful and at worst counterproductive, potentially creating negative associations and otherwise disrupting what truly should be a fun, stress-free parenting win.

This simple framework is how I developed a literacy-promoting environment for my own daughter. Starting from our first days of life, we began flipping through the pages of the books gifted to us at my baby shower. At two months we introduced a bedtime story as part of her nighttime routine. Reading became second nature, as frequent and expected as diaper changes and feedings. My husband and I placed board books in every corner of the house, in every room and on every play surface. It made playtime fun and easy: Sitting in her bouncer, she would babble and smile as I read to her, handing over *Goodnight Moon* so she could explore and chew on the pages. By nine months, she crawled and cruised on her own, and used reading as a pit stop between play mats. One of her first words was "book," which she repeated to me as she brought a story over and backed up adorably to sit in my lap.

Creating an early reader was a definite parenting win. It was something that I knew was important, that I could easily promote, and that made me feel like I could tangibly affect and improve my daughter's development. Get ready to feel this same parental empowerment.

THE BOTTOM LINE

5 out of 5 Pediatrician Parents Agree

- Early literacy is important because it promotes normal infant development—including language and motor skills, bonding and physical touch with parents, and stimulating all of baby's senses.

- No need to compete over which baby can tackle Tolstoy fastest, but there are indeed long-lasting effects to early literacy like earlier language acquisition and enhanced cognitive performance later in school.

- Promoting early literacy is insanely easy: place books around the house, incorporate story time into routines (like bedtime) starting in the first weeks of life, and view board books as a fun toy to incorporate into play.

- The best books (and toys!) for your baby are the ones that *you* enjoy. Babies are captive audiences and will like whatever story you read to them—so find some classics that you don't mind rereading early on. Making sure that you have fun during story time will make you want to keep at it.

13

TV LAND

● ●

Screen Time Isn't Actually Baby Poison

I was pregnant and had my baby during my pediatric residency. Having just turned thirty, I still considered myself young and hip enough to stay up-to-date on the newest trends in technology. For my teenage patients, this meant knowing how Snapchat was being used or which instant messaging platforms were trending. For babies, it was all about two words: "screen time."

During my training, the world of official, pediatrician-sanctioned screen time recommendations was quickly evolving. Back in 2015, the sentiment was simple: Screens are bad. The American Academy of Pediatrics recommended strict avoidance of visual contact with literally any type of screen (video chat, tablet-based activities, you name it) for kids under two years of age. Then suddenly, on a child's second birthday, they magically gained the mental capacity to handle up to two hours of screen contact every day.

The backlash was expected and appropriate. With no compelling evidence to justify this restrictive approach, many pediatricians joined parents in asking the AAP to create realistic recommendations that acknowledged the complex science behind baby screen time. Previous ultraconservative screen time guidelines were based on shaky data. For example, a famous study linked sedentary behavior (including but not limited to watching screens) to childhood obesity. As always, correlation does not equal causation. It's hard from an ethical perspective to do a randomized trial and make a bunch of infants binge-watch Netflix while the others have a screen-free childhood filled with developmental activities. The associations we find are certainly multifactorial. As one example, toddlers who watch TV programs with commercials for unhealthy food products may have an obesity-risk increase simply due to this targeted advertising, rather than the duration of screen exposure.

So after taking a hard look at the data (including new studies showing that video chatting with family is important for social connection and actually provides more benefit than harm), the AAP did agree it was time to make some important—if small—changes. The new-and-improved 2016 AAP policy still bans solo, passive screen use until eighteen months, at which time parents may introduce no more than sixty minutes per day of "high-quality, educational" programming. But the key difference is that this recommendation doesn't include "constructive or connective" screens like video chatting, taking photos, making videos, looking at maps, or searching the internet to find information.

These AAP rules were generally held as doctrine throughout my residency, and I'm grateful my training finished before the infamous 2019 WHO guidelines—suggesting a complete ban on screens for the first two years of life, followed by a strict sixty-minutes-per-day limit from ages two to five years—came into place. Because even with these somewhat more realistic recommendations, it seems that screen time rules are still being created in a vacuum.

It's why even as a pediatric resident I had trouble reciting AAP screen time gospel verbatim. A child of the nineties, I had watched more than my fair share of television during my formative years. When parents asked me for advice on introducing screens, I suggested that they do their best to stick to the official recommendations but acknowledged that a one-size-fits-all approach to parenting (or anything) is never the right approach. I distinctly remember when one single mother, who worked full-time and shuttled her two- and four-year-old daughters back and forth to day care every day, literally laughed after I suggested limiting screen-based entertainment to one hour daily. "Do you know what my morning looks like?" she asked good-naturedly. God bless her honesty. She said she'd do her best to reduce tablet use and TV time. But wasn't it better for everyone to use screens as needed to maintain a consistent, relatively calm morning routine?

With covid, it seems the world is starting to catch up to the privilege inherent in these unrealistic expectations. I remember the summer of 2020 like it was yesterday, when #PandemicParenting brought a whole new meaning to the phrase "good enough parenting." As all parents struggled, it was clear that the impossible challenges of working parenthood during a certifiable plague were not distributed equally.

One day in July, as I doom-scrolled through social media, I stumbled upon a thread filled with blog posts and essays from parenting experts now compelled to repent their promotion of screen time abstinence. These parents were newly faced with the task of being the primary caretaker of their children (while working from home, of course, and without nannies or preschool to provide engagement and entertainment). It became immediately clear to so many how the benefits of some screen indulgence outweighed any risks, pandemic or no. It was an important moment for me. Not only did I feel infinitely better about the role that Baby Shark and Doc McStuffins were playing in my daughter's chaotic, covid-era upbringing (it was a sizeable role), but I was more confident than ever that my realistic screen time counseling had always been the right approach.

Even though I was a few years ahead of my time in my "try your best," screen time preaching, when my daughter was born, I unfortunately did not extend the same kindness and reason to myself. Instead, my anxious brain latched firmly on to the hypothetical negatives of screen use. And steering away from so-called perfection, even as I counsel others to embrace life's realities, isn't something that comes naturally to me. If there was a chance of harming my baby's beautiful neurons and preventing her from reaching her full cognitive potential, why on earth would I risk it? My secret goal was clear: keep my baby from as many dangerous screens as possible, for as long as possible. At the very beginning, we often had TV on in the background as she slept in our arms, with the sounds of an *Arrested Development* marathon hopefully indistinguishable from ambient conversation. But as she got older and less inert, starting to look at the world around her, we generally didn't have the TV on or put her in front of screens at all. For a few months, a relatively screen-free existence (at least when my daughter was in the room) was sustainable.

But my daughter quickly transformed into an increasingly alert and demanding infant. For the most part, it was easy and fun to entertain her. In some instances, however, it was clear that using a screen had a whole lot more benefit than risk. Years before the pandemic uprooted our collective sense of work-life balance and childcare crises, and even in very privileged circumstances, there were plenty of times when my husband and I were left scrambling to keep our jobs, care for our infant, and get the bare minimum of sleep to drive into work the next day. For example, when my nanny got sick and I had to take care of my six-month-old at home by myself between two night shifts, I felt that if I didn't get at least a little bit of rest I might actually die. Desperate, I exhaustedly placed my phone streaming YouTube children's videos in front of her bouncy chair and slept on the couch next to her. Two hours of fitful sleep later, I was able to make it back to the intensive care unit for another night of work.

My daughter seemed to emerge from her screen time "binge" unscathed. I took it as a sign to finally be more realistic and even more permissive. Screens are a part of our lives, and my daughter will grow up in a society where they will impact her day-to-day functioning. It is simply a fact that all children will need to learn how to interface with screens in many forms. Wouldn't it be nice if we had some recommendations that not only acknowledge—but also embrace—this essential truth?

Let's dive into my evidence-based approach that minimizes the risks of excessive screen exposure without creating unrealistic expectations. When parents ask me how many hours of screen time is acceptable, I resist giving a numeric answer, and instead recite these *Ten Screen Time Commandments*:

1. **Not all screens are created equal (some are inherently better than others).** It's important to think about how screens are used and what content they can deliver, but some screens are just going to be better than others in almost any context. Trust your instincts. After years of restrictive guidelines, blog posts, and even outright shaming, it's all too easy to get caught in the trap that anything with a "screen" is automatically evil. For example, an interactive tablet designed for babies (V-Tech, etc.) is much more like any other electronic toy than a fully functioning screen. A tablet that streams Netflix and YouTube videos, on the other hand, is basically a TV. It makes sense, but it's easy to get swept up in the hysteria. Playing with electronic toys, letting your baby explore your e-Reader (which is much more like a book than a true screen), or pressing on a touchscreen menu can essentially get free passes.

2. **Abstinence is impossible.** We live in a world where screens—of all shapes and sizes—are omnipresent. Unless you go completely off the grid, there is a 100% chance your baby will have significant exposure to screens before their eighteen-month birthday. It's much easier to control a baby's screen exposure if you embrace it.

3. **Less is more, but counting screen time minutes in that first year probably doesn't make sense.** The magical eighteen-month cutoff, where one hour of screen-based "entertainment" becomes suddenly safe, is based on nothing. Sure, we know that those early months of a baby's life are crucial for development. And yes, it certainly tracks that minimizing time with eyes glued to a screen will allow for all the important developmental activities a baby needs. There is science, and it does support the idea that less is more. Young children who are exposed to screens beyond AAP recommendations have been shown to have differences in brain structure, as well as changes in language development and sleep, for example.

    The biggest problem with these studies is that they are all observational, and so many other factors are likely at play (absence of other developmental activities, access to early literacy, nutrition, and socioeconomic status, just to name a few). Certainly, a good portion of the effects we see are because of these other associations. In the age of covid, we know now more than ever that a screen-free or limited-screen existence is a marker of privilege.

The other problem with using these observational studies to support strict time cutoffs in screen recommendations is that they are designed the exact opposite way you'd want them to be. It's nothing that the researchers did wrong, it's simply another limitation of this type of study design. The only way to truly know what a "safe" amount of screen time is would be to take a bunch of babies and randomize them into groups where they get different daily screen exposures (zero, twenty minutes, forty minutes, an hour, etc.). This is, for obvious reasons, unethical, and would be logistically challenging regardless. This means that our information relies on parents reporting how much screen time they allow kids to consume. Not only is this potentially inaccurate (I can't remember how much *Pete the Cat* my daughter watched yesterday, let alone last week), but it also oversimplifies things. Current studies tend to divide children into two groups: those who consume more than the AAP recommended amount of screens, and those who don't. This means that those studies showing language delays, brain changes, and other screen-induced woes have had to group very different situations together. For example, an infant with four hours of TV-time daily would be in the same category as one with twenty minutes of daily screen use.

In the end, the science is real and there is data *suggesting* associations between screen use beyond AAP recommendations and developmental issues. Screen time moderation and cognizance is certainly important. But the reality is that there is no magical time limit that will assure your baby is free from the potential deleterious effects of screens. It's far more important to embrace all the other measures that help use screens in their appropriate and appropriately limited contexts, and forget about tracking your baby's minute-by-minute screen consumption.

4. **The most, most important part of a screen is *how* it's used.** There's an enormous difference between sitting a six-month-old in front of a tablet to solo-watch *CoComelon* on Netflix and having a parent physically sit next to them and use that very same tablet to play an interactive game. Having a parent and baby touch a screen together introduces a whole world of fine motor, social, language, and even gross motor skills.

   It's really *restrained* screen time that's the biggest problem. The observational studies showing increased risk in obesity, social issues, and sleep problems all look at sedentary screen use. So watching *CoComelon* on TV while crawling around on the floor and chewing on stuffed animals is a

213

different experience for a nine-month-old than doing so while buckled into a bouncer.

It's yet another reason that you shouldn't worry so much about time limits. Shorter stretches of low-benefit, sedentary screen time seem safer, but I view them as more harmful than longer stretches of higher-engagement screen-based activity. I'll vote for a rainy afternoon snuggled as a family on the sofa with a full-length movie over a daily, strictly limited thirty-minute session alone with a tablet any day. How both parents and children engage with screens—and each other during screen time—matters more than anything.

5. **Stay skeptical of "educational" programming.** Yes, as a pediatrician, it's the law that I love *Sesame Street*. But Rule #4 always wins, even for high-quality public broadcasting. While I would have *loved* to drop my daughter into her ExerSaucer and fall asleep to the dulcet background noise of *Mister Rogers' Neighborhood* on particularly nap-inducing rainy days, I did this sparingly. Instead, I favored turning on my beautiful infant's beloved and insipid *Baby Shark* videos so we could dance and sing together. In short, the "educational" value of a show doesn't undo the ill effects of nonstop, solo, physically restrained screen use.

6. **Sometimes, the rules don't apply.** There will be times when the benefits of using a screen—even

a passive one with insipid programming—will be greater than the benefits of stubborn abstinence. When kids are in the hospital, we give them whatever tablets they need to get through poking and prodding, helping them feel as safe and comforted as possible. Plane rides are survival of the fittest, and I will keep letting my daughter watch unlimited movies using her adorable headphones for as long as this entertains her (you're welcome, everyone else on our flight). Don't martyr yourself. I promise that the misery from hours of screaming (especially in situations—like long flights—that you can't escape) is much worse than some extra screen time.

It doesn't even have to be an extreme situation. There will absolutely be days when work has been exhausting, life is too stressful, or something is just sapping your last ray of loving, attentive energy and you simply need a break. It's okay for YouTube videos to tag in as the nanny to get a few minutes' of rest or an extra half hour of me time.

7. **View screen time as negative space.** Don't forget: Passive screen time spent watching programming on tablets, phones, and televisions is often replacing time that would have previously been spent on more hands-on interactivity. Think about it: If a six-month-old watches hours of YouTube videos each day instead of playing with caretakers, doing tummy time, practicing holding

and reaching for objects, etc., it makes sense that a delay might develop. That is to say, it may be less about the addition of screens into our lives and more about what they are replacing.

If most of your baby's day is spent reading books, playing with caretakers, exploring the world around them, and engaging in other developmentally stimulating activities, there's no need to stress about letting them watch a whole movie (gasp!) one morning so that you can nap for an extra hour.

8. **Practice what you preach.** This was (and remains) by far the hardest rule to implement. It's relatively easy to monitor a baby's daily screen exposure, but your own? All parents, like all modern humans, are to varying and increasing degrees slaves to technology. There's nothing like trying to minimize your baby's screen time to make you realize just how insanely screen-filled your life is.

Recognizing the role of personal screen use is just as important as any other technology regulation for babies. The time that we spend checking our email or scrolling through social media is time away from our little ones. Sure, we all need some alone time, and if that needs to take the form of a screen binge, that's more than fine. But the key is cognizance. Being aware of this more insidious and passive screen activity is in many ways more important than any other screen regulation. These moments bring all the bad of baby screen exposure—distraction from human interaction, replacing developmental activities— with essentially no real benefit. Other than, as I mention, the very real and important benefit of keeping a technology-dependent parent sane! While there's no need to ban all adult screen use around infants, just realize that it's another messy part of the equation. Setting some boundaries is helpful—for example, pushing yourself to keep phones away from the dinner table, or scheduling an hour of strict screen-free family time each evening. In the end, modeling reasonable screen behavior from the beginning will help you set the tone for how you want your family to interface with technology as your little one grows.

9. **Video chat gets a free pass—at least until we invent holograms (or teleportation).** The AAP is okay with FaceTime and other video chatting, and so am I. Studies show that the social and emotional benefits of staying connected with family not only neutralize the "risks" of screen exposure but also likely outweigh them. How could anyone deny the importance to the entire family of showing grandparents, friends, and family how your infant is doing and enhancing these bonds over geographical distances? As I'm sure no one needs reminding, the pandemic has made spending time physically together in the same room harder

than ever. My toddler and I FaceTimed friends and family for hours each day that we were stuck in strict quarantine during the spring 2020 New York covid surge. There was no doubt in my mind that the benefit of virtual interaction with other children was enormous compared to any potential risk.

10. **Set yourself up for success.** Strict time limits may be so 2016, but it's okay to have some restrictions. Creating healthy boundaries and even some ground rules is a good way to make sure you don't let the passive onslaught of screens take over your baby's life. This might be some simple interior design—like facing the TV away from your dining area and committing to sit-down mealtimes, even when your child isn't around.

    I like to view the issue of screen time less as a daily one and more as a week-to-week. If we go three days with no TV, then indulge in a rainy-day movie marathon, I don't sweat it. But if our work and childcare situations are relatively stable, and it's been a few days in a row of more than an hour with Netflix as the nanny, I make a mental note and try to make some scheduling changes for the rest of the week.

THE BOTTOM LINE

5 out of 5 Pediatrician Parents Agree

- Screens are ubiquitous in the modern world, so it's time to embrace them. Focus on how to make your baby's screen exposure healthier and set expectations you can meet.

- Less is more, especially in the first year. Time limits are based on weak studies, so you can worry less about a strict hour-per-day rule (or even complete zero-tolerance ban) and think instead on a week-to-week daily average.

- Not all screens are the same. Interactive screen use, snuggles on the couch while watching a movie, and especially video chat like FaceTime are entirely different beasts than strapped-in, solo YouTube viewing.

- Screen time is usually negative space. Find balance by shifting focus as much as possible to promoting the activities that screens tend to replace—reading stories, playing on the floor, cruising and crawling, screen-free family meals, etc.

- Some situations are survival of the fittest. At the doctor's office, on a plane ride, or even after a long day of work when you just need a few moments of rest, indulging in the occasional, unlimited screen orgy is more than fine.

14

BILINGUAL BABY

• •

Why It's Totally Great to Raise Your Baby in Whichever Language(s) You Choose

The American child is a linguistic anomaly. Around the world, speaking a single language is a rarity, and it seems that our increasingly globalized society is finally realizing the benefits of raising a polyglot. But surprisingly, the topic of if, how, when, and why to expose infants to multiple languages remains controversial. I've seen parents who are still reluctant to raise their baby in a truly bilingual household, worrying that speaking multiple languages at home will cause speech delay. Others, whose anxieties are enhanced by the predatory baby product market and competition among their parent peers, are desperate to enhance their child's linguistic ability, spending money and stress on classes and products that probably don't work. While there is a role for promoting language learning in the first year of life, the majority of activities and products available for sale are costly and unnecessary. I've seen plenty of parents spend needless time, money, and worry on tutors, language systems, or day care "enrichment" classes only to be deeply disappointed when the result is anything less than complete fluency.

Let's walk through the most common language acquisition questions that I hear.

Should I Raise My Baby in a Bilingual Environment?

The first, fundamental question is simple: Is it worthwhile to raise a baby with the goal of fluency in multiple languages? In short, yes. Multilingualism is about more than "just" opening doors to different cultures, careers, and opportunities later in life. In fact, studies show that learning languages as a baby seems to provide children with a completely new way of thinking, opening their minds not only to different languages, but also different logics, literally changing the structure of their brain. Children who speak multiple languages have enhanced executive function (problem-solving and attention), do better on tests of social skills, and demonstrate higher levels of emotional intelligence. Bilingualism may even protect against dementia in older age, and researchers in Canada found that their bilingual Alzheimer's patients performed much better than expected on tests of memory and problem-solving than would be predicted by their amount of brain atrophy.

I've always taken it for granted that multilingualism is a goal to aspire to. Yet I still meet many parents who are concerned about the risks. Parents hear that babies exposed to multiple languages develop speech delays, but in fact the evidence is unclear and inconsistent. Even where there is supporting data, the delay is always temporary; there's no indication that raising a baby who is exposed to multiple languages puts them at a developmental disadvantage in the long term. Some worry that having a child fluent in a language they as a parent are not fluent in will create a communication barrier, but this is also a myth. Babies quickly learn who in their lives understands which languages, and effortlessly, instinctively choose the correct language for each listener. Multilingualism is an asset—not a roadblock—in developing communication skills.

This is what I told Hannah's parents when I found out, at her one-year-old checkup, that her parents, who were from Japan and spoke English with an accent, were limiting the amount of speaking they did when she was in the house. Their friends had explained that speaking to Hannah in Japanese-accented English would negatively affect how she herself learned English. Online, they had come across endless horror stories of children raised in a non-English-speaking house and how this had translated to delayed speech and poor preschool performance. What choice did they have but to leave her language development to the experts at day care and not cause any harmful confusion?

Hannah's story isn't simply a cautionary tale on the perils of pseudoscience and misinformation. It's an extreme that shows how a little bit of science and common sense is all you need as "permission" to speak to your babies in your own native language. Communicating with your little ones should be fun and intuitive—not a chore.

Raising a Bilingual Baby Is an Admirable Goal. How Should I Do This?

Once you embrace that raising a baby with multiple surrounding languages is a good idea, the next question is, logically, how? If you speak a second language at home, or have caretakers who speak a different language, this is an easy task. But what about parents (like me!) who speak only one language natively?

Some brief background: If I hadn't become a doctor, I would have without a doubt been a linguist. I still wistfully recall my college days in academic paradise, sitting in a foreign language classroom conjugating verbs and reviewing the subjunctive. (I know, I'm the epitome of coolness.) But after years of study, I was only ever passably fluent in two languages—in addition to my native English, I had a good amount of exposure to Spanish as a child and studied it intensely in school. I can still speak proficiently, and this ability has been the singularly most useful skill in my career. It also set me up to place outrageous expectations on my parenting. For years before I was even thinking about having a baby, I ranted to friends and family that I would do whatever it took to raise a child who was fluent in Spanish. Even before we started trying to conceive, I researched local bilingual day cares, and casually asked around for native Spanish-speaking nanny recommendations. I had made a promise to my unborn child, and I refused to go back.

For the first nine months of my baby's life, we had an incredible nanny who spoke "only" English. So to provide my daughter with true multilingual exposure, I bought books in Spanish, played Spanish music, and did my best to speak to her only in Spanish when it was just the two of us together. But while the books and music were fun for everyone, forcing myself to speak my non-native language during my limited free time to play with my daughter was ridiculous. My grammar was clumsy and my vocabulary was limited. It took me months before I realized that speaking to my daughter in my own language was more than okay, and I was still a good mother providing her with an enriching and nurturing environment.

Please, learn from my mistakes. There's robust science that shows why torturing yourself in order to provide language lessons isn't just stressful, but also less useful than you might think. This is because babies become bilingual through immersion, and only through immersion. Those books in Spanish, that music, those mommy-and-me classes I didn't have time for, are simply a fun way to expose your baby to new sounds and cultures. Babies can't learn from Duolingo or Rosetta Stone; those classes and interactive videos are worth only as much time and money as the enjoyment they provide. The reality is that unless a main caretaker is speaking almost exclusively in another language, a baby will not be bilingual.

When Do Babies Need to Be Introduced to Languages In Order to Become Fluent?

When I say that a baby will not be bilingual without immersion, what I mean to say is that a baby will not be bilingual *yet*. The mastery of language and how those brain connections change does depend on when a foreign language is introduced, but deciding the exact cutoff age for each degree of language fluency is quite complicated. There's evidence from the lab that important stuff is happening in those first weeks of a baby's life, with connections between sounds, words, meaning all at their most malleable. But while there may be theoretical benefits to exposure right from the newborn period, we know that most of those positive, brain-shaping effects can still take place later on. Language learning is complex, dynamic, and there is even a brain-imaging study that showed adolescents had similar changes in brain structure whether they started learning a language at birth or later in childhood.

While the debate still rages among sociolinguists and behavioral psychologists, the practicality is that children will be able to speak fluently, without an accent, as long as language immersion begins before the teenage years. In other words, there's absolutely no need to stress about language exposure in that first (or second, or even third) year. There will be plenty of time later to enhance your child's linguistic ability.

When my daughter was almost one year old, we moved to a new state and hired a nanny who spoke limited English. My daughter spent most of her days hearing only Portuguese, and the result was a gorgeous, linguistic mess. My daughter's primary language is English, but she also clearly understands Portuguese. I often spoke to our nanny in Spanish as a sort of lingua franca, and I naively thought my daughter didn't understand what we were saying. I was wrong. Planning a day's activity with my nanny is almost impossible in front of my daughter now that there is no safe language to talk about "friends," "the park," or "ice cream" without her immediately making demands.

I have no idea which language(s) my daughter will be fluent in—or even which ones she already is. But once I decided to truly go with the flow and view language development as something

that would happen naturally (and based on my daughter's sur-
roundings), I was able to view my role in my daughter's language
acquisition less like traditional homework and more like Spanish
grammar workbook homework—that is to say, super fun.

As a piece of parting advice, I will add that if you have the
opportunity to expose your child to multiple languages, take
advantage of it. Like Hannah's parents, I've seen an unexpected
number of families who choose not to provide a multilingual
environment even when it's available. The reasons are varied,
and it seems that the concern for language confusion and speech
delay underlies most of this decision-making. I've met countless
nannies in educational classes, story times, playgroups, and
other enrichment programs who have confessed that they are
not allowed to speak in their native language to the children
they care for. The irony seems to be completely lost—having
caretakers bring children to educational programs while reject-
ing the built-in language tutor in your house is illogical.

The truth can set you free. Rather than agonize over language exposure and linguistic development, you can simply let
everyone who cares for your baby—yourself included!—speak
whatever language makes it easiest to enjoy your time together.
While early multilingualism is definitely not harmful—in fact,
it has long-lasting brain benefits—it's nothing to stress over.
The solution is simple: Speak to your little one in whatever lan-
guage(s) let you most easily share love and affection, which is
what your baby needs most of all.

THE BOTTOM LINE

5 out of 5 Pediatrician Parents Agree

- Multilingualism is great for brain development—and does *not* cause meaningful speech delays—so if exposure to foreign language is available, you should absolutely embrace it.

- Babies only learn language through immersion. Those mommy-and-me Spanish classes and baby Duolingo can be fun, but they won't turn your little one into a polyglot.

- Immersion means immersion. A caretaker who is fluent in another language must almost exclusively speak that language for a baby to be truly bilingual.

- If you can't immerse your infant in a foreign language before their first birthday (or second, or third . . .), there will still be time to become bilingual.

- Language learning should be fun. All caretakers should speak in whatever language they feel most comfortable in, letting them be as talkative, engaged, and interactive as possible—which is what matters more than anything.

PART THREE

6 to 12 Months

15

BABY TEETH

• •

Everything You Need to Know about Teething and Oral Hygiene for the Smallest Smiles

I love the dentist. Not like, love. I'm the rare human who genuinely looks forward to her dentist visits, adoring the feeling of professionally scrubbed teeth so much that I've never missed a checkup. In my first year of pediatric residency, the only day I had off for months coincided with my birthday. I was delighted and scheduled my routine cleaning on that same day as a present to myself. So when the office where I saw my patients in residency began its dental health initiative, boosting our counseling to patients and teaching us how to paint fluoride onto baby enamel, I was in heaven. I also vowed to remember all these brilliant recommendations when I had my own baby, and give her the brightest, healthiest smile a child could have.

My expectations were ambitious. After my daughter cut her first tooth, I diligently brushed her tiny tooth nub every morning and every night. I placed a rice-sized drop of strawberry-flavored, fluoridated toothpaste on the finger brush, laid my daughter in my lap, and meticulously scrubbed her little nub with what I imagined was the devotion and attention of a dental hygienist. My pediatrician mentors would be so proud! It was easy and fun. Then one day, after a few weeks, my baby decided she was done cooperating. I was on a busy rotation in residency, leaving the house by six a.m. almost every day and spending many nights sleeping over in the hospital. With her enthusiasm waning, and my exhaustion waxing, strict dental hygiene became a lesser priority in the months to come.

Until I saw a cavity. One morning, as we were finishing our snack of fruit salad and getting ready for a stroll outside, I saw grooves in her molars that looked like gaping black holes. My heart raced—had my dental neglect led to early childhood cavities? Cavities this young are rare, and usually indicate trouble with a baby's genes, diet, or overall care and hygiene. I brushed her teeth twice that night and called the dentist for an appointment the next day. When she came home from day care that Monday, I looked again—they were now gone! I recalled the fruit salad ingredients and was both embarrassed and relieved. The discoloration was from blackberries, and those apparently gaping holes were peels that had stuck into her grooves.

After the blackberry incident of 2019, I tried to step up her dental routine at least a little bit and made every effort to brush twice daily. After my daughter turned one, she began enjoying "teeth time," learning the phrase and demanding her toothbrush whenever we passed the bathroom.

Even without my own dental angst, it can be hard to decide how much to worry over your baby's tiny teeth in the first year.

In a world where being a "good parent" comes with an impossibly long list of responsibilities, the emotional and physical capacity for parenting tasks is more limited than ever. Let's go over how to protect your baby's smile without losing your own.

I spent years telling parents that they had to scrub their baby's teeth just right, that the crying and fighting was worth it, and that there was no excuse for a missed session. The sentiment is on point, and doing your best to stick to twice-daily brushing is an admirable goal. When cooperation is an issue, there are certainly ways to make "teeth time" easier. The internet is filled with awesome tutorials from seasoned pediatric dentist parents who will patiently demonstrate strategies for efficient and effective infant dental care. But it's also a reality that even the most diligent, patient, and dentally enlightened parents will see some days, or even weeks, where strict twice-daily brushing falls by the wayside.

When the struggle kicks in, remember that your best is enough, and that you're also doing lots to protect those tiny pearly whites in ways you might not even realize. It turns out that the most important ingredient to maintaining healthy smiles is a balanced diet. Maintaining sugar intake in moderation (no need to eliminate completely, though, as we'll review later in Chapter 17) will keep almost every child free of tooth decay. Some sugar is worse than others: Anything that pools on teeth—like sipping on a bottle of juice or putting sweeteners on pacifiers—has extra potential for damage and is something you can eliminate altogether. In the end, doing your best to stay on top of "teeth time" and focusing on healthy eating is usually all you need to do to promote a cavity-free childhood.

What about the other items on the full list of infant dental recommendations you'll find on official and decidedly unofficial guidelines alike? Besides nutrition and earnest attempts at twice-daily brushing, another way you can protect your baby's enamel is topical fluoride. Feel free to go ahead and buy the fruity-flavored baby toothpaste that comes *with* fluoride right away! I still see a huge amount of outdated advice online suggesting that fluoride-free toothpaste is the only safe way to go until your baby can spit out toothpaste on their own. But this is simply not true. A rice-grain-sized dab of toothpaste that you brush onto your infant's teeth is safe, even if they swallow a good amount of it. And it's effective at preventing cavities, especially for babies who are at higher risk. Fluoride tablets, on the other hand, have gone completely out of fashion, even if you use water from a well or other fluoride-free source. They're no better than topical treatments, can cause discoloration of enamel, and are a pain to remember to take.

The last box on your infant's dental hygiene checklist? Deciding at what age a dentist wants to see your baby in their office. The American Academy of Pediatrics recommends setting up that first visit right away, as soon as six months if a baby's first tooth has popped up. The American Dental Association generally agrees, recommending a visit by age one or within six months after a baby cuts their first tooth. I agree that scheduling a dental appointment on your baby's six-month birthday is an admirable goal, but as I know all too well, a trip to the dentist often loses priority over more pressing issues. I still adore dental checkups, and I would never discourage a timely visit before your baby's first birthday. There's lots of important counseling to be done, any serious issues can be detected and treated early, you may get some fancy fluoride varnish, and it will boost a positive relationship between your baby and that often-dreaded but actually amazing dental chair. Nevertheless, if life gets in the way and that first visit slips into your baby's second year of life, focusing on "teeth time" and a balanced diet will assure that both their health and your own sanity stay intact.

Next, it's time to prepare for the stress that baby teeth can cause even before they're visible. There are endless teething myths, and I've seen how often legend—spread by family, friends, parenting blogs, and message boards—prevails over science. Let's set the record straight with a fun game called Myth vs. Fact: Teething Edition.

1. My baby is crying all the time because they're teething

Likely "fact." Teething is a leading cause of serious baby fuss, and it's not uncommon for babies who are cutting teeth to spend days or weeks crying much more than their usual. It's very reasonable to blame some extra meltdowns on emerging enamel, but remember that it's not the only possibility. Teething gets an understandably bad rap, but we do tend to blame more baby discomfort on it than is often the case. The first year of life is filled with coughs, colds, sleep regressions, accidents, and all sorts of potential reasons your little one might be in a particularly bad mood. Most of the time, it doesn't matter what's causing the discomfort as long as it's manageable. But if something feels off, if your little one just won't stop crying, or you are concerned for any reason at all about their behavior, call your pediatrician to troubleshoot and make sure there's no need to investigate a little more.

2. My baby's fever is because they're teething

"Myth," at least by technical definitions. Because the first year of life is filled with those fuss-inducing cough and cold viruses, it's also filled with the fevers they cause. Viruses are by far the most common cause of fever in infants, and a true, sustained fever is most likely to be caused by an infection. There's evidence to support this, with studies failing to show any compelling relationship between teething and fevers.

Many parents, and even seasoned pediatricians, still swear that teething can cause temperature elevation and even "mild" fevers. It makes sense that there could be an increase in body temperature with teething; we know that teething causes inflammation, something that greatly influences temperature. Some of the confusion also has to do with what we consider to be a "true fever" in infants (100.4 degrees Fahrenheit), and what any elevated temperature that doesn't pass this threshold even means. Most of the "low-grade" or "mild" fevers we see don't pass this cutoff, bringing us back to where we started: that "real" fevers are caused by something besides teething. And all pediatricians agree that sustained, "true" fevers are much more likely to signal an infection. If there's any confusion, just ask your pediatrician. The answer may be as simple as a prescription for extra cuddles and some social distancing.

3. **My baby's congestion, runny nose, rash, diarrhea are all because of teething**

Mostly "myth." To expand upon our theme, the most common cause of congestion, runny nose, diarrhea, and rashes in infancy are those same viral illnesses that cause the fevers we can't seem to stop blaming on teething. Babies get random rashes all the time, have all sorts of random poop changes as they explore new foods, sniffle and sneeze for no reason, meaning there are plenty of other explanations for why a teething infant might have some combination of these symptoms. Some of it could of course be related to the inflammation we see in teething, but again the data seem to point toward viruses as the main culprit. In the end, it doesn't matter all that much. Your happy, snotty, rashy baby likely doesn't need much more than the TLC you're already giving. And when in doubt—yes, you guessed it—call your pediatrician.

Now that we've set the teething record straight, let's dive into the burning treatment questions I hear from parents daily. I'll help you ignore the harmful remedies and focus on the real treatments that will help teething be as pain-free as possible.

Are There Any Medicines That Can Help?

Tylenol's a good option! Acetaminophen (the generic name for Tylenol) is an extremely safe medication in babies with no serious side effects. It usually provides better pain relief for babies than adults, so if you're like me and almost never find it helpful for yourself, just know that it's probably soothing your baby's aching gums significantly. After the age of six months, babies can have ibuprofen too, another safe pain reliever that is also anti-inflammatory. If you find that your baby constantly needs these medications, however (especially both in combination), remember to check in with your pediatrician and make sure there isn't something else causing extreme fuss and discomfort.

What Else Works?

The best remedies for teething are the simplest. You can ditch fancy tinctures and ointments (more on that next) and place some wet washcloths and teething toys in the freezer instead. A cold or frozen, safely chewable toy or cloth is the most effective and safest option. Add in some snuggles, a lot of patience, and plenty of parental self-care, and I promise you'll get through even the worst teething fuss as painlessly as possible.

Do Over-the-Counter Herbal Teething Drops Work?

No, return them! Trendy, "natural" solutions are worse than ineffective—they're incredibly dangerous. How dangerous? These remedies are completely unregulated. Most teething drops contain benzocaine, a numbing medicine, which even in small amounts can prevent baby's blood cells from carrying oxygen—leading to serious damage and even death. Other "alternative" drops contain an unregulated amount of plant-based chemicals. One "naturopathic" teething tablet contained so much belladonna (a heart-stopping plant used as poison) that at least ten infants died from using it.

Those Amber Teething Necklaces Look Great, Where Can I Get One?

Don't do it! Amber teething necklaces can also lead to tragedy. In 2018, the FDA reported multiple reports of infant injury—including two deaths—directly from using these horrific choking hazards. Just remember: When it comes to aching gums, the simplest solutions (cold washcloths and toys, Tylenol and Motrin if needed, and a whopping dose of TLC) are the safest, most effective way to go.

THE BOTTOM LINE

5 out of 5 Pediatrician Parents Agree

- When your baby's teeth come in, do your best to brush them twice a day with fluoridated toothpaste.

- The most important step in keeping your baby's teeth healthy is to avoid excessive sugar, especially anything that pools on their teeth—like sipping on a bottle of juice or putting sweeteners on pacifiers.

- If you have the bandwidth, schedule a visit with the dentist in your baby's first year. This will help your family get used to the dentist and get some helpful tips and anticipatory guidance. But if life gets in the way and seeing the dentist slips off your to-do list, it's okay to just focus on avoiding sugar and brushing as best you can.

- Teething myths are myths. Try not to blame your baby's inevitable fevers, congestion, rashes, and diarrhea on their emerging enamel.

- Tylenol, cold cloths, and frozen teething toys are all that your baby needs to get through cutting teeth. Necklaces and drops are dangerous, and you should simply avoid them. If Tylenol and toys don't cut it, call your pediatrician—chances are, your baby has something else going on.

16

NEVER WAKE A SLEEPING BABY

∙∙∙

Myths and Facts about Bed- and Naptime

Is it true that "sleep begets sleep?" Is it okay for babies to nap more than expected for their age? What about napping less? Should you change a baby's natural nap routine? Are there any harms from letting a baby nap all day? Are strict nap schedules a good idea? Infant sleep (or lack thereof) is one of the most stressful topics for new parents. It seems that more time is spent discussing sleep habits than getting a good night's rest during that chaotic first year of a baby's life. Even parents who have diligently sleep trained, cried it out, or otherwise figured out a recipe for getting their little ones to (mostly) stay quiet through the night can feel like the worry never stops.

It's an (unnecessary) stress I know well. During the first months of my daughter's life, I never could have imagined complaining that she was sleeping too much. At four months, we won a short but hard-fought battle with sleep training, and I could not have been happier. At nine months, our family made the move from Michigan to New York, an exciting

241

but exhausting process that completely changed everyone's routine. In the two weeks between moving and starting my new job, I stayed at home with my daughter for some quality bonding, unpacking, and setting up our new life. It was wonderful to get to spend so much time with my baby, but it was a big transition. The move meant having to leave behind our Supernanny, who had jointly cared for our daughter and my friend's son, since our daughter was just a few weeks old. Both babies had seemed to take morning and afternoon naps at almost the exact times each day. They were changed, fed, played with, bathed, and smiling no matter when we walked in the front door. I assumed, having only one baby to care for and as a competent mother, that it would be easy to translate this routine seamlessly to our new life. A sample schedule lovingly written by my Supernanny in hand, I woke up our first Monday in New York ready to run back the Michigan playbook.

It took a mere two hours for my plan to go off course. At nine a.m., my daughter was due for a morning nap. She screamed, clearly awake and wanting to play more. I obliged and tried again each hour until finally putting her down successfully at noon. At three p.m., I still heard gentle snores. Should I wake her? Worries popped into my head, both reasonable and outrageous. Would letting her sleep later mean she would have trouble falling asleep at night (reasonable)? Was sleeping this long a sign of a serious neurological problem (outrageous)? Would just one long nap give her as much energy for the rest of the day as her usual two (reasonable)? Would skipping a nap permanently stunt her brain development (outrageous)? I was weeks from sitting for my pediatric boards to certify my expertise in all things related to children's health, and I had no idea if my daughter's napping was normal.

As we transitioned to our new routine over the next few weeks, her sleep schedule continued to transition as well. Some days she took two short naps, some days one long one, some days two naps so long that I had trouble pushing aside the thought that something might actually be wrong with her. My pediatrician-mom friends reassured me, but I couldn't resist consulting the internet. Big Mistake. It was clear that whatever I was doing was bad. It's crucial, the internet advised, that babies have a strict nap schedule. Actually, it was terrible to have a nap schedule and caretakers should spend their entire days asking babies if they are ready to sleep and only put them down when they say "yes." One nap was okay in this age group. Actually, one nap was not okay in this age group, and my baby's exhausted brain would have problems forever. Didn't I know that babies in Finland nap more than American babies and that's why they are so much smarter? It was day three of my brief stint as a stay-at-home mom, and I thought I was already failing.

Pediatricians understand much of the complex neuroscience of sleep in babies, countless sleep disorders, the general amount of sleep a baby needs, and overall trends in baby napping. We often explain the expected infant nap schedule to new parents in a quick one-page handout. This chart will show you that for the first month or so, your baby will essentially almost always be asleep, with on-and-off naps taking up around sixteen hours of their day. Infant sleep needs decrease gradually, and each month you'll likely see your baby sleep just a little bit less each day—meaning they'll likely still be asleep more than half of the time by their first birthday. What changes most, however, is when they get that sleep. While a newborn will split their sleep pretty evenly between day or nighttime (or even exhaustingly save their most alert times for the middle of the night), a six-month-old can often sleep ten to twelve hours overnight, saving the rest of their sleep needs for a nap (or two, or three) during the daytime hours.

But despite the leaps that pediatric sleep science has made in recent decades, there are still surprisingly few official, pediatrician-approved answers to more complex nap questions. It's why even as an almost-board-certified pediatrician, I was overwhelmed by unscientific, unhelpful, unrealistic, and endlessly conflicting advice—preaching strict nap schedules, waking sleeping babies to make sure they're tired for bedtime, or banning sleep-scheduling altogether.

It's time to replace nap charts with nap philosophy. Get ready to ditch one-size-fits-all sleep guides and instead embrace a few basic principles that will assure that your baby gets the sleep they need without making you lose any yourself.

Sensible, Scientific Infant Sleep FAQ: Pediatrician-Mom Edition

Does Your Baby Need a Nap Schedule?

No. There's no evidence to support the idea that babies on firm nap schedules are somehow healthier than those whose nap-times are more flexible. Think about it: What are the chances that, over the course of human history, normal development was dependent on a fixed sleep schedule in infancy? It's exceedingly more likely that our species, instead, evolved under circumstances where parents let babies take their naps at will—or whenever they fit into an already busy schedule of basic survival.

Do YOU Need Your Baby to Have a Nap Schedule?

Almost certainly. A strict napping routine is indeed a modern, made-up worry. But we also happen to live in a modern world. Around three to six months, when all this talk of schedules starts to come front and center, also happens to be when most parents are either back at work or settling into a stay-at-home parenting routine. Even the most easygoing caretakers need some structure to build their day around. Whether it's being cared for by a nanny, at day care, or at home with mom or dad, it's the rare situation where some basic naptime plan isn't helpful. So while there may be no developmental need for a baby to have a stringent nap schedule, there are definitely benefits to caretakers creating some discrete sleep times.

How Do I Make a Nap Schedule?

It should come as no surprise that the honest—if frustrating—answer to this question is "it depends." All babies are different, with temperaments and sleep needs that make prescribing a strict one-size-fits-all nap schedule impossible. And all families are different in their scheduling needs, adding another fun, complicating layer to the sleep-scheduling challenge.

But I'm not here to throw you to the proverbial wolves. It's hard to know what your family's particular naptime routine will look like, but the steps to get you there are easy to predict.

1. **Try not to worry too much about nap schedules at all until your baby is three months old.**

   For the first months of your baby's life—lovingly called "the fourth trimester"—they will behave in many ways more like they did in utero than they will as they grow into an alert, human infant. It's a product of our biology, with all babies being born a little less "cooked" than most other species and needing even more care than you'd expect someone who's already been evicted from the womb to need. Your baby slept whenever they wanted in utero (and often during the day, when the movements of an awake, pregnant parent rocked them to sleep). During the fourth trimester, your baby will demand these exact same lazy Sunday-esque vibes. If your nesting period allows, keeping naptime super chill and schedule-free for the first three months or so is going to be the easiest way to let everyone get the sleep they need.

   In a society with woefully inadequate parental support, however, most families (at least in the United States) will find themselves unable to go without some sort of sleep schedule for this long. It's impossible to have an honest discussion without embracing parenting privilege, a topic that comes front and center any time we touch on the social support necessary to minimize stress as a new parent. If having a rough schedule much earlier than the three-month mark is necessary to go back to work, transition to a new caretaker, or just survive life with a newborn, that's okay too. The younger your little one is, the more challenging it will be to get them to follow your naptime lead. But it's not harmful to try as long as you follow some basic cues and aren't consistently keeping them awake when they're tired.

2. You're the expert in your baby's sleep needs.

As a parent, you're the boss of your family, and the expert in your baby's needs. Full stop. This means that you are the best person to decide when the task of creating a sleep schedule is worthwhile for the structure it provides. And it also means that you know better than anyone else how much sleep your infant requires.

I mean it. You don't need a PhD in the neuroscience of infant sleep to figure out if your baby is getting enough sleep or not. Those nap charts—and check-ins with your pediatrician—are a great start. But remember, you've been watching your baby sleep their whole life! You know their evolving sleep trends, the cues that they're tired, or the happy, alert play signaling a nap well-taken. You'll be able to use these patterns, combined with the reality of your own day-to-day routine, to create a general sleep schedule that fits everyone's needs.

3. Stay flexible—as much as you can, at least.

Ever had a day so exciting that you couldn't fall asleep 'til midnight? What about an exhausting day that had you passed out on the couch by eight p.m.?

Infants, like every adult I've ever met, would answer "yes" to these questions if they could. There will be plenty of times when your baby, no matter how easily they go down for a typical nap, is just not able to stick to whatever routine you've created. And that's okay. Expect to have the (at least) occasional "off" day, whether it's because your baby was too tired to stick to their routine, because you had to adjust it for a special event, or simply because your childcare fell through and you just couldn't pull your act together at home. When "off" days become patterns, it's often because there's a naptime transition point approaching. Is your baby tired all the time and can't make it to their next nap? Maybe a nap was dropped a little too soon. Consistently fighting that morning nap no matter what you do? Could be time to consolidate and shift the schedule. Keeping attuned to their cues, and responding to the patterns you see, will assure that your little one gets the necessary amount of rest to grow and thrive.

Is It Okay for Babies to Nap More Than Expected for Their Age? What about Napping Less?

In short, yes. Averages are averages, a concept we will talk about in great detail in Chapter 18, and an elusive truth that leads to needless parenting stress. And just like infants instinctively know how to eat (which we'll explore in Chapter 17), they also know how to sleep. We've been doing a bad job of giving babies credit for the (relatively few) things they are in fact able to do expertly. Regulating their own sleep needs—and letting you know if you're doing an okay job of letting them meet these needs—is something they are in fact awesome at doing.

I repeat: Babies are born to autoregulate sleep. If you give them adequate stimulation when awake, let them sleep when tired, and don't consistently force them to stay up when they'd rather be snoozing, there's no biological concern that they will be sleep deprived (or somehow over-rested). And remember, who's driving the ship is key. There's a big difference between a baby who is constantly woken up from naps to fit an overstuffed schedule of activities and a baby who wakes up on their own from short naps because that's what their body craves.

Even when childcare realities alter your little one's "natural" sleep patterns, you'll be able to adapt. When my daughter started day care, I panicked that the shorter, less frequent nap schedule would turn her into a sleep-deprived baby zombie. But it ultimately worked out just fine. Depending on her nap-needs du jour, she was able to take a rest in the "cozy corner," nap during our commute (thanks, New York City rush hour traffic!), or doze at home before dinner on the couch.

If you still find yourself stressing over how much sleep your baby is getting, remember that a quick call to your pediatrician will outsource the worry and sort through things in no time. And if your infant is "lethargic," seems impossible to wake up, or has any change in activity that just doesn't seem right, let us know! Serious problems are rare—the most likely explanation is an undetected virus that needs some extra snuggles—but as always, there's no need to triage on your own.

Does "Sleep Beget Sleep?" Should I Never Wake a Sleeping Baby? Is My Baby's Bedtime Too Late? How Can I Be Sure My Baby's Sleep Schedule Is Really Okay?

Deep breaths. With endless sources of information, advice, and feedback, you might still find yourself needlessly doubting the expert, bespoke sleep routine you create for your infant even after reading (and rereading) the road map above. I went through it myself. Settling into my own nap- and bedtime routine with my daughter meant not only debunking my own pediatric worries, but also facing countless questions and judgmental comments on sleep patterns (and the schedules we made for her).

Tune it out. Any guidance that you find should be used only as much as you find it helpful, and only if it's something that you can customize to fit your family's evolving needs. There's simply no magical number of naptime hours that will allow your infant to grow, develop, and reach their full cognitive potential.

An additional pro-tip: being tired is the enemy of sleep. It's why so many parents find that the solution to super-early morning awakenings is counterintuitively to push bedtime even earlier. I'm a huge fan of this as well, with plenty of personal and professional success stories. Does that mean there's anything inherently "wrong" with raising your infant as a night owl? No, and there are parents who favor a later bedtime, have babies who still sleep through the night, with the whole family still getting enough sleep and staying well rested.

Getting good rest—whatever that looks like for your baby—is the key to a successful sleep schedule. It's why I do agree that "sleep begets sleep," however your little one interprets that rule. So just like most babies do better with a bedtime routine that starts earlier (usually when they're less tired), they often do better with an uninterrupted afternoon nap. I don't think it's fair to say you should "never wake a sleeping baby," but we can dispel the myth that allowing a baby to nap too late will disrupt bedtime. I can personally attest to an extreme example of this not being true, with my daughter frequently napping up until just an hour before bedtime—and still going to bed as easily (and sleeping as long) as usual. As a rule, getting a good night's sleep has more to do with how parents put their babies to sleep and much less with when their naps end (check out those bedtime routines we talked about in Chapter 10). Stay attuned to the patterns you see and embrace a whole lot of trial and error. I promise you'll be able to find a schedule that works for you, recognizing the strategies that work (or don't) for increasing your little one's restfulness.

THE BOTTOM LINE

5 out of 5 Pediatrician Parents Agree

- Nap schedules aren't strictly necessary. As long as babies are allowed to sleep during the day when they are tired, they will grow and develop just fine.

- But we live in a modern world. Having a schedule helps all caretakers—stay-at-home parents, nannies, and day care teachers alike—get through the day's activities. A general timetable provides a consistent routine that benefits everyone.

- Your nap schedule can be as strict as you want, but be mindful that babies are people and will have different sleep needs day-to-day. And if you need to change naptime for an awesome activity that sparks joy for you both, that's totally okay too (and can help your baby become a little more flexible as well).

- Some swear that waking their babies up during naps helps them sleep better overnight. Others push bedtimes to try to help babies sleep later. Every baby is different, but in general, sleep truly does beget sleep. Earlier bedtimes and uninterrupted naps tend to make bedtime easier and let little ones get longer stretches of overnight sleep.

- Babies know how to sleep. If you are responding to your infant's cues, letting them sleep when they're tired, and creating a sleep schedule that meets both of your needs, your little one will grow and develop just fine.

17

LET THEM EAT CAKE

• •

How to Introduce and Sustain a Healthy Diet without Excess Restriction, for Good and Picky Eaters Alike

Dinnertime! After months of milk, you'll eventually find yourself looking at the solid food menu, ready to share meals with your baby. As with everything else, there is plenty of confusion (and way too much stress) about how to start your baby's solid food exploration. I'm here to explain the actual science behind infant nutrition so you can choose a safe, convenient, and personalized approach that fits with your family's unique preferences and values.

Let's dig in!

When Should I Give My Baby Solid Food?

I was taught to tell parents that the answer to this question is "six months." And while this is a solid answer, it's helpful to understand why this recommendation holds water. For most of modern history, deciding when it was safe for a baby to consume anything other than milk was based primarily on our understanding of their physiology. In the first months, babies don't have the motor skills to eat solid food, which requires some basic physical ability that nursing or bottle-feeding does not. Like being able to keep one's head and neck upright, having strong enough jaw muscles to mash even soft purees, then tongue strength to push it down the esophagus, then a coordinated swallow mechanism that gets food safely into the stomach. It's why through the 1990s, it was common for pediatricians to let parents introduce solids as early as three to four months—as long as babies had developed these necessary skills.

But it turns out it makes sense to wait even longer. In 2003, the World Health Organization published new and improved guidelines based on studies showing that exclusive breast-feeding through six months of age correlates with substantial health benefits including lower obesity rates and fewer infections. It's unclear whether this correlation is related to introducing solid foods later, or if it might have more to do with the positive effects of breast milk. What we do know is that the first few months of life are critical for baby gut development, especially the crucial "good bacteria" (remember colic theories in Chapter 8?) that are important in protecting against a variety of gastrointestinal ailments later in life. It doesn't mean that the absence of solid foods (and/or the presence of more breast milk) are the direct *cause* of these intestinal benefits. But it does give biological plausibility to the theory that waiting to interrupt a baby's belly biome causes some physical changes that make future stomach problems less likely.

We also have evidence that delaying the introduction of baby food may have other benefits. In 2016, scientists in the United Kingdom surveyed thousands of families and found that babies who didn't eat solids until age six months or later were less picky as toddlers, refused food less often, and were less likely to be diagnosed with a "feeding difficulty." It's counterintuitive but helps put to rest fears that waiting too long to introduce flavors will create a less adventurous eater. It's weirdly the opposite. Some hypothesize that older babies have the motor skills to try foods with different flavors, and that's certainly possible. But it seems the better explanation is that, in general, parents who wait longer are also the same parents who (overall) promote positive eating habits. Newer research has found lots of connections between the early introduction of solid food and other behaviors that can lead to obesity (like regular intake of juice or soda before age two, for example).

It's complicated, to say the least, and all of this convoluted data reminds us that what matters more than anything are the patterns in our parenting decisions rather than any choice we make at a given point in time. All these feeding choices— even the "simple" decision about what day you'll give your baby their first savory solid morsel—are just part of the bigger picture. Your family's relationship with food is what ultimately matters more than anything else. So none of this is make-or-break, and if there is some personal, logistical, cultural, or any other reason that giving solid foods before your baby is exactly six months old makes sense for your family, it'll be okay. For most families, though, waiting until this cut-off makes sense, so hang tight!

Which food should I start with?

Every once in a while during my three years of residency training, I'd listen to a lecture that was genuinely fun. Baby nutrition was always a good one. Our presenter, a seasoned pediatrician and experienced mother, passed around purees, puffs, and yogurt bites to taste. Trying not to hoard the sugary-sweet morsels, I listened as she turned to the room for some Q&A-style teaching. Her first question to the group: What do we tell parents to feed their babies once that six-month birth-day arrives? A few hands shot up: pureed something, canned something—anything Gerber? Rice cereal is also a good way to go. The presenter waited—any other possibilities? My col-league, the only mother at the time at that point in our train-ing and a quiet genius who you always wished would speak more, raised her hand. She had done "baby-led weaning" with her children and had read about its safety and benefits. Did the lecturer ever counsel families to try this?

The answer, to my surprise, was yes. Many of my class-mates were shocked. For decades, doctors have been telling families to take a stepwise approach to introducing solids, starting with pureed and bland items, and then progressing slowly to harder but still "baby-friendly" foods with a limited number of ingredients. It surely makes sense that an infant with developing oral-motor skills and no teeth can't eat a car-rot, and throughout history, parents have boiled, pre-chewed, or otherwise softened those first bites to help their babies learn to eat. But the idea that infants can only have a very limited number of "baby-approved" first foods is relatively new and coincides with—surprise!—a booming baby food market (estimated at $77 billion in 2021!).

When the first patented baby food came on the market in 1921, the idea was to take advantage of canning and preserving technologies to provide a product that would free American mothers from manually boiling, mashing, and pureeing their infants' meals. When profit ensued, formula companies like Gerber quickly hatched a plan to create a parallel movement for solid infant food, capitalizing on the sentiment of the time that "scientific" products were inherently better than anything a mother could provide. It worked, and commercial baby food soon became ubiquitous, championed as a product that wasn't just safe, but in fact superior to homemade infant meals. By the 1970s, decades of ingenious marketing had created an entire philosophy of baby nutrition. Parents— and doctors—existed in a world where giving prepackaged and "baby-safe" foods was the expectation. It's what television, radio, and even pediatricians told families their infants needed.

The 1970s and 1980s saw mothers pushing back, and in a world where automatic blenders made mashing meals into mush a less athletic feat, more families began preparing their own baby foods in earnest. Still, it hasn't been until the past few decades that an even more fundamental discussion has taken the stage. There's really no need for commercial, prepackaged baby foods, and the sugar, salt, and preservatives make them on average less healthy than home-mashed meals.

But *what*, exactly, is the best food for a baby's first bites? And how do babies get to the point where they can eat the same dinner as their parents?

Plenty of pediatricians still encourage parents to use blended purees and cereals. It's also what many trusted parenting guides still tout. At six months, baby can have a single-grain boiled cereal spoon-fed to them as they sit strapped into their high chair. At eight months, feel free to introduce a few pureed fruits and vegetables. At nine months, try a mashed avocado, banana, or other single-ingredient soft food. After that, start slowly introducing other soft finger foods or spoon-fed mashes, one at a time, and don't venture more boldly until baby is one year old.

I absolutely recited a regimen almost identical to this one as a training pediatrician. But that fateful lecture, where the words "baby-led weaning" were first introduced into my brain, changed my thinking forever. The general concept of baby-led weaning is a pretty great philosophy. Instead of shoving rice cereal into a baby's mouth, you place the soft foods that appeal to them—a smashed banana, avocado, mashed potatoes—at your baby's reach, or offer it (but don't force) via a spoon. Babies still need food to be a little softer, but there's no magic to boiling, chewing, straining or otherwise smushing fruits, grains, and veggies into baby-friendly servings. No ingredient restrictions (except honey, but that's a rule that prevents infant botulism), and no more pressuring baby to eat when they aren't hungry. Here comes the airplane, open wide? Not anymore. Instead, here comes the healthy, balanced mealtime, where everyone sits at the table together and regulates their own hunger, exploring a varied and delicious menu.

When my daughter turned six months, I was already committed to—and excited about—this approach. An unenthusiastic cook before new mom exhaustion further decreased my motivation, I couldn't imagine spending hours preparing purees or spending money on cans of sugary cereals. Perhaps a little too eager, we gave her a piece of quesadilla. She spat it out, confused. Fair enough. We smashed a banana and mixed it with breast milk. Delicious! Over the next weeks, as her chewing improved, we branched out: avocados, eggs, hummus, cooked carrots, even bites of mild enchiladas we got for takeout. We watched her carefully, avoided choking hazards, and followed her lead. It was simply a blast.

Sharing banh mi with a seven-month-old still sounds insane to plenty of parents. But baby-led weaning really isn't so radical. It's still about starting with softer items and slowly progressing to more texture. Rather than following a strict timeline and restrictive menu, however, it lets babies decide when they are ready to move on to the next phase. It makes a whole lot more sense than pretending we know the exact age at which each baby is going to be ready for the next stage of food exploration. It also teaches babies how to know when they're hungry. Yes, it's just a correlation, but we do have research showing that infants who undergo baby-led weaning are on average less likely to be obese than those given traditional baby foods.

While there isn't anything wrong with giving babies some canned purees or prepackaged snacks if it makes your life easier—in general they have more sugar than home-cooked meals, so moderation makes sense—staying flexible with feeding makes mealtime easier and more fun. My own experiences solidified the real benefits of the baby-led weaning approach. For example, I saw my daughter more quickly develop the fine motor skills needed to pick up food; not spoon-feeding her meant we could sit down for meals together and develop a routine, and she sat happily in restaurants while we split eggs benedict for brunch. In addition to these perks for social and motor development, it made adventurous eating the norm, and is one of the key techniques to stave off the picky-eating habits of early toddlerhood.

In the end, I've seen lots of success with using baby-led weaning as a starting point. Like everything, you'll need to adapt to your own needs, and your mileage may vary. Some parents have much more time (and patience) to sit with their little ones and watch them explore their mushy menu than others. And plenty of families find that their own day-to-day reality (including having other caretakers who may not be able to put in the time and effort) makes it impossible to stick to the baby-led approach. So if and when some spoon-fed purees and sugary pouches make it into your little one's diet, don't sweat it. Modify as needed, and ignore any one-size-fits-all advice that comes your way.

How Can I Get My Baby to Actually Eat These Foods?

It's true, all toddlers will experience some degree of "pickiness," so it's important to understand that having a one-year-old who loves kale salad as much as you do is not the best goal. But my baby absolutely could find plenty she liked on a sushi menu, at an Indian restaurant, or any outing of our choosing. The truth is that baby-led weaning did most of the heavy lifting. By her first birthday, my daughter had sampled more dishes than I could count. Shrimp tempura? Check. Peruvian chicken? Check. Pad see ew? Check.

Baby-led weaning gives infants the chance early on—when tastes are developing—to experience a rich and varied diet. Countless studies on infant feeding prove that tiny babies will try anything. The window for maximum adventurousness seems to be between six and nine months, sometimes up to a year-old. Taste isn't even a factor, and six-month-olds really will sample whatever you put in front of them. Taking advantage of this window of culinary exploration can reap huge benefits. And sharing your menu and time at the table together also means that mealtimes are social. Eating becomes fun, not a chore.

Here's another elusive, essential truth: Babies don't have "tastes," they just have moods. Decades of research has shown that it often takes even dozens of tries before a baby decides that a food is worth chewing and swallowing. My daughter refused chickpeas six times before they became her favorite food. One week she would eat more avocados than I had in the house, only to refuse them the next week. There's no way to know what a baby will want to eat on any given day, at any given meal, at any given second. So just keep trying, and the rest will be what it may be. You can't control what your baby eats, you can only control what you offer. Results may vary, and even promoting adventurous eating from the very first bite doesn't guarantee your toddler won't binge on chicken nuggets and mac-and-cheese for a week at a time. But the combination of some sort of modified baby-led weaning, offering varied and healthy choices and keeping the stress out of mealtime, will prevent picky eating from becoming patho-logic. With this approach, you can rest assured that as long as your baby or toddler is growing, they will be absolutely fine.

I can't stress enough how important it is to set the stage for a positive eating experience early on. As a hospital pedia-trician, I've treated more than my fair share of toddlers who can't gain weight—and even need feeding tubes—because they simply refuse to eat. It's called an oral aversion, and usu-ally happens when kids were sick early on and developed bad associations with being forced to eat. But this extreme gives credence to a common-sense philosophy: forcing a kid to eat can have long-term consequences.

What's love? As the great Ashanti once said, "It should be about trust." The greatest lie of modern parenting is that "expert" strangers know more than you do about your child. And a very close second is the myth that we parents know more about our baby's bodies and instincts than they do. An infant's skill set is extremely limited, but it absolutely includes knowing when they're hungry, when they're full, and being able to use this information to take in the nutrition they need. No matter how you decide to feed your baby, there will inev-itably be a time when you feel, for whatever reason, that you need to teach your baby how, what, and how much to eat. No need to be hard on yourself when that moment arrives—but no need to indulge it, either. Allowing your baby to regulate their own hunger and nutrition means letting go. In the absence of providing an all-day Oreo buffet, the risk of over-feeding your infant when they signal for more is nil. Same goes for underfeeding, especially in the first year when breast milk and/or formula still make up the bulk of their nutrition. I can't count how many times my daughter went on an almost twenty-four-hour solid-food strike, only to consume what appeared to be at least three thousand calories of fruit, veggies, pasta, eggs, and whatever else I was eating next to her the following day. Baby-led weaning only works if it's actually baby-led, and focusing on quantities rather than the overall relationship your family has with food is the easiest way to turn a fun parenting win into a counterproductive struggle.

Is It Okay to Have Dietary Restrictions for My Baby?

Next, it's time to explore what that healthy menu looks like for infants. Let's dispel a few hard-held myths about baby nutrition necessities. The biggest is that there is a one-size-fits-all menu you must embrace, and that your family's dietary restrictions are verboten for your infant. Your baby can absolutely join you in your pescatarian, kosher, halal, vegetarian—and yes, even vegan!—diets. This remains a highly controversial topic in pediatrics, with doctors understandably worried that restrictive diets will deprive little eaters of crucial macro- and micronutrients. For this reason, plenty of pediatricians still prescribe dairy—and sometimes even meat—as absolute musts. But science doesn't quite support that. The thing is, we still don't understand what adults are supposed to eat!

As the dieting fads cycle between plant-based/vegan to all-meat/no-carbs and back again, it's clear that even scientists are often guessing. Doesn't it make more sense to figure out what molecules in food are needed for kids and build up from there?

I remember Alex, one of my regular office patients who was back to see me for his nine-month visit. He was growing and developing beautifully, and since there were no vaccines at this age, it was a leisurely appointment, a time to catch up and answer questions. His parents had started solid foods and were loving baby-led weaning. We went over the foods he had explored, and what was next on the menu. When I asked about yogurt and cheese, his parents' faces changed. "Well, they began, we're both vegan and haven't been able to bring ourselves to give those to him yet." They had chosen this diet for ethical and health reasons, and even though they had been told how important it was to give dairy, it was an emotional challenge. It just didn't feel right. I paused. I knew the traditional advice, and understood its reasoning: Giving Alex cow's milk would be an easy way to ensure he was getting enough fat, calcium, and vitamin D. But there are plenty who argue compellingly that feeding kids milk from a different species is, well, weird. Cautiously, I ventured back into the conversation. Did they want Alex to be vegan?

Their faces lit up, and I sensed excitement and relief. Of course that is what they wanted, but only if they could do this in a way that didn't sacrifice his health. I told them the truth. They could, but it would take a little more work. Developing baby brains depend on a diet full of fat, and since vegan food is still targeted at adults, recipes would have to be altered and high-fat foods prioritized. Calcium and vitamin D come to kids in recommended doses through fortified cow's milk, so this would also have to be planned out (a daily vitamin could help too and would prevent him from becoming deficient in iron and B-vitamins usually obtained from meat). Did they want to meet with the nutritionist to come up with a meal plan? They did.

You too can work with your pediatrician and pediatric nutritionist to come up with a menu that matches your baby's needs and your family's values. The truth is that almost all dietary preferences can be tailored to provide infants with the nutrition they need.

An important caveat: Baby-led weaning, with whatever dietary preferences your family decides on, is only healthy if you share nutritious foods. Studies consistently show that how healthy a family eats at home is the best way to predict how healthy a kid will be. It's not about restrictions. Simply having nutritious options available and providing a varied menu is all you need. It's what sets the stage for years of good eating, appropriate weight gain, and overall well-being. You can rest assured that allowing your baby to share Ollie's celebratory cupcakes at day care won't undo all the hard-earned benefits of a healthy at-home diet. In fact, steering away from overly stringent dietary rules is one of the most important ingredients to providing your little one with a balanced relationship with food. And what the science consistently shows us is that it's just as important—if not more important—to focus on how you frame access to sweets, treats, and assorted processed goodies as it is to make sure they're consumed in moderation.

The mantra of moderation is a great way to make sure that eating is as nourishing to the body and mind as possible, and that it stays that way. Only you will know what the ideal menu looks like for your family, based on whatever combination of personal, ethical, religious, and cultural principles matter most to you. And only you will know how strictly you want to extend those preferences to when your child is outside of the home. You'll want to make sure that you've done the right amount of reflection—and research—to help you decide what food convictions you hold, and why they are meaningful to you.

The most common source of confusion I see around this is when it comes to the "clean" food craze. Food science is a real and evolving field, and it's taken me years to gain an even basic understanding of what all those healthy-sounding buzzwords even mean. There's a steep learning curve, and you'll want to read up on the most up-to-date expert musings on the environmental nuances of different types of agriculture, the equity issues with "organic" farming, and why the "non-GMO" label is almost always a marketing ploy. I know you'll be able to sort through it all and come up with a meal plan that matches your moral values.

Just remember to keep that healthy dose of consumer skepticism, and know that sticking to a low-stress, moderation-centered approach (especially at those cupcake-filled birthday parties) will have more health benefits than anything else. It's easy to get swept up in the idea that anything without a leafy-green label is harmful. We do, after all, live in a world where "clean" wine (which is still chock-full of toxic, liver-failure-inducing, cancer-causing alcohol) is somehow made to feel like a healthier choice than "artificial" infant formula.

But we also live in a world where environmental toxicity is very real, and a very real threat. It's certainly reasonable to try to reduce this exposure to your baby when you can— as long as the benefits of doing so are based on real science and don't create more stress than they need to. For me, this meant focusing a lot less on food labels and just doing my best to strive for variety. The reality is that the dose makes the poison, and the easiest way to minimize exposure to any toxin—be it "natural" or lab-made—is to ingest less of it. I paid attention to broadening the culinary options available to my daughter instead of eliminating certain ingredients based on limited and questionable science.

Just over a year after Alex's visit, I met him in my office for his two-year checkup. He was a rambunctious and adorable toddler, with parents who had been able to provide nutrition in a way that was consistent with their values and without sacrificing his health. In the end, this is what all parents want, and it's completely achievable.

THE BOTTOM LINE

5 out of 5 Pediatrician Parents Agree

- Plan on waiting to introduce solid foods until six months.

- Baby-led weaning is great, and you can absolutely give your baby normal human food from the beginning. Foods need to be a little softer at first, but your baby will decide which textures they are okay with. Avoid choking hazards and go ahead and share your takeout meals right away.

- "Baby food" is fine if it's convenient (those yogurt pouches and puffs are portable for picnics), but most of them are much less healthy than sharing a sliced banana or giving plain Cheerios.

- Baby-led weaning is only healthy if *you* generally eat healthy food. Focus on stocking a pantry full of good food choices. If you offer a balanced menu to your baby, they will eventually get a balanced diet (on their timeline, of course!).

- You control what your baby eats and when your baby eats. Your baby controls if they eat and how much they eat. If your baby is growing, they are getting enough food.

- Junk food and treats are fine in moderation, but being too obsessed with "healthy" foods can turn mealtime into a chore. Birthday party cupcakes and ice cream socials have more benefit than harm.

- A balanced diet looks different for every family. There are no rules for which exact foods babies need, and they can share any dietary restrictions their families do—even veganism. It just might take a little extra work to make sure they get all the micro- and macronutrients they need, so talk to your pediatrician.

18

MILESTONE MADNESS

●●●●●●●●●●●●●●●●●●●●●●●●●●●●●●●●●●●●●●

Nurturing Development without
Unnecessary Stress

Baby's first steps! Baby's first word! It seems every pediatrician's office and social media feed can't stop talking about developmental milestones. But how obsessed with "meeting milestones" should you really be? In this chapter, we'll take some time to understand why pediatricians use developmental milestone cutoffs at all, how we interpret them, and how much (or little!) you need to stress over them. With some science and common sense, you'll be able to enjoy every "first" without undue angst, while still assuring that your little one grows and thrives at their own perfect pace.

Milestone anxiety is a worry I know all too well. My daughter was born one month premature, but to my delight, she met all her early milestones on time, and I couldn't help but feel proud that she was already "catching up" to the babies born at term. Then came walking. My daughter was one of the rare children who do something known as "knee scooting," a term that came to my attention after endless nights in the depths of Google searches and parenting blog posts. At ten months old, my daughter had discovered that instead of crawling on all fours, she could lift her arms and trunk and move around on her knees. Soon, she could move faster on her knees than she ever could crawling. Walking was new, balance was hard. Why wouldn't she continue with an efficient and safe method? It was adorable, quirky, and smart.

Until it wasn't. At around twelve months old, my pediatrician brain started screaming. I had just finished my residency and passed my pediatric board examination. That meant that in the prior few months I had been studying development and memorizing (just like I had been since my second year of medical school) the expected ages at which babies start to do the things that babies do. Things like smile socially (two months, check!), coo or babble (four months, check!) sit up (six months, check!) cruise, crawl, or pull to stand (nine months, check!) and walk (twelve months . . . baby, the test answer is twelve months, did you hear me?). I reassured myself that those were just averages, expected ranges, and babies are all different. I knew I had to wait.

I pushed more flashcard images out of my head over the next few months. It was hard not to feel like we were working on a deadline. Then one beautiful spring day, as my baby knee-walked happily around the house with a smile, I felt my heart racing. She was now fifteen months old, the age where not walking is officially a "red flag." My daughter was . . . *delayed*. I talked to every one of my friends, the pediatricians and non-pediatricians alike, seeking out reassurance that my unique knee-scooter was healthy and normal. I reread all the blogs. There was relief: @firsttimemama12 went through the exact same thing with her daughter, who at seventeen months old started walking and never stopped! But then, more panic: @papabearneedscoffee thought his adorable knee-walker was totally fine, until the pediatrician ordered an X-ray that showed abnormal hips. No wonder baby Jack didn't want to stand!

I don't blame myself for being obsessed—nor do I blame other parents! Milestone madness is *everywhere*. While I decided against taking photos each month of my daughter posing next to a sticker with her age, my social media pages were full of these, each post listing the child's developmental accomplishments. My pregnancy app, unused for months, flashed frequent notifications asking me about my baby's first smile, coos, and movements. At every routine checkup with my pediatrician, I filled out the same screening forms I had so often interpreted for my own patients. Could my daughter pass a Cheerio from one hand to the other? Would she find a toy that I hid in a cup? Did she smile and laugh consistently? How frequently did she look at an object I pointed to? Every answer that wasn't a resounding *yes* gave me pause and put me even more on edge.

Reaching developmental milestones can feel like a never-ending process of checking boxes these days. But the reality is that infant development is its own complex, dynamic, evolving science. Before we decide if, when, and how much to worry about each box that goes unchecked, we have to take an important step back. Here's a brief primer on the stages, domains, and framework we as pediatricians use to understand child development in all its exciting, messy glory.

When baby experts talk about an infant's development, we divide their achievements into "gross motor," "fine motor," "language," and "social/problem-solving." Tables and charts abound, but there's no need to dive into each and every milestone unless you're studying for your pediatric boards. The broad strokes are what matter. For gross motor development, your baby will start their life able to wiggle their body but not much more. They'll progress to holding their own head up around two months of age, rolling over at around four to seven months, sitting up around six to eight months, and taking their first steps usually around their first birthday. Their fine motor skills will also be initially unimpressive, but they'll start to hold objects around two to three months, bring things to their mouth with their hands around five to six months, and by twelve months might even start to hold objects with their cute little clawlike finger grasp. Language is completely receptive at first, meaning your baby will just start by processing gestures and sounds. As they grow, they'll start to make singsong vowel noises that mimic conversation (cooing, around four to six months), and then singsong consonant noises in a speechlike pattern (babbling, around seven to nine months). And they'll get pretty clever and friendly pretty fast. For the first few months, they won't be able to follow your face or voice consistently, or even smile when they're happy. After their social smile around two months, however, they'll quickly learn to laugh, giggle, blow cute little spit bubbles, mimic your sounds, know your scent, prefer you over strangers, play peek-a-boo and other games, and respond to their own name in their first year of life.

It's always good to be prepared, and knowing what to expect in your baby's first year will help you set up your home and your day-to-day living in a way that keeps your little one safe and helps them explore their world. Part of the "anticipatory guidance" your pediatrician will review at each checkup will be exactly that—reminding you of the milestones your baby is likely to achieve soon, how to foster their growth, and how to make sure you have a safe setup for their ever-increasing mobility.

But milestone madness has become about so much more than productive preparation. These ranges of motor, social, and language development have started to feel like deadlines. It's hard not to want to ditch developmental monitoring altogether, throw those Instagram milestone blankets and blocks in the trash once and for all, and ignore all the checklists, pediatrician assessments, and anxiety-provoking vigilance that comes your way.

The struggle is real, but I promise there's a middle ground—and a reason that laid-back milestone monitoring is important for your infant's health (and can even be a fun parenting experience!). The main purpose—besides anticipatory guidance—of tracking your baby's developmental progress is that some delays predict problems later on or indicate that another medical condition is the cause. As a pediatrician-in-training, I assumed that all milestones mattered in this way. But in fact, this isn't the case. Researchers in the Netherlands recently published a study looking at the dozens of developmental milestones that pediatricians track in the first four years. They found that out of seventy-five milestones measured, delays in only nine of them predicted problems functioning later. The ability to predict problems was significant but small. What was more significant? *Combining* milestone measurements. A single delay is unlikely to predict a real problem. It's when a baby has multiple delays—generally the delays that cross different domains, like social, speech, fine motor, and gross motor— that causes seasoned pediatricians to worry.

Pediatricians and assorted baby development experts are always trying to find better ways to detect meaningful delays without adding unnecessary anxiety. But we know it's a work in progress, and acknowledge plenty of limitations in the templates, checklists, screening forms, and handouts we use. Sometimes, it's just that we collect "too much" data without providing enough context. *We* know that we don't usually need to do anything other than keep watching when our forms come back with red flags. If there's an isolated delay, we rarely do more than watchful waiting or a referral to early intervention, where physical, occupational, and/or speech therapists will decide if any extra support will provide a developmental boost. We know that even most "meaningful" delays will correct themselves with time, with that early intervention boost, and don't act as harbingers of developmental badness to come. Fully understanding the framework and rationale for all our developmental screening is the most important part of removing the stress of pediatric milestone monitoring.

But there are also important, intrinsic limitations in the creation of milestones themselves. When we take a step back and understand where cutoffs come from—and what data there is to support them—it becomes clear that these milestones are ranges that should be interpreted carefully, applied to each situation individually, and should be used only as a tool to help developmental progression and not to "grade" it.

Where do these "norms" even come from? It depends on which source you use, but there are two main ways that professional organizations (like the CDC, WHO, and AAP) use science to define "normal" pediatric development. The first is by having experts take years of experience and whatever data they have available to come up with cutoffs. More guidelines than even most pediatricians realize are created with this type of methodology, and the CDC and AAP milestones are the most famous examples. Where data is limited or lacking altogether, there's been some good faith effort to conduct studies with large groups of children to see if the milestones these organizations put forth are backed directly by science. Other developmental assessments do have a good amount of evidence behind them, and many newer screening tools that specifically look for delays (rather than just give expectations and norms) were created based on large sets of data, using fancy statistical modeling full of fun words like "mean," "standard deviation," and "Gaussian distributions."

In either scenario—whether an organization's developmental "norms" are based directly on large data sets or validated later with studies—the end result is often a list of the average age at which babies achieve specific developmental milestones. And after a few games of data-interpretation telephone, this gets translated into what parents are told—on every chart, in every parenting book, on every social media feed—is "normal." If you see a single number (babies roll at four months! They sit up at six months!), chances are that this number is based on the age at which 50% of babies reach that milestone. It's a useful number for the people who study infant development, but not a particularly useful number for any one baby or parent. For example: Say you and your daughter are in a playgroup of ten six-month-old adorable little rascals. Since the milestone for sitting up without any help comes at six months old, it could seem at first (as it does to many, even many pediatricians) that most or even all of them should be able to do this. But that's not how percentiles work—rather, by the law of averages, that playgroup should have only five babies who can do this. That means five perfectly happy, normally developing babies may very well have parents who are worrying about a *delay*. Yet the weirder finding would be a room full of babies who can all do every single thing that half of six-month-olds can do.

Okay, so unless you're studying for your board exams or conducting your own developmental research, there's no use for milestone averages beyond the basic anticipatory guidance they inform (and that your pediatrician will be all over). But isn't there some point at which a milestone is delayed enough to cause worry? Pediatricians have a cutoff age for when a baby's failure to reach any given milestone is a "red flag" and cause for some alarm—or at least a little extra vigilance on our part. These "red flags" are sometimes based on expert opinion with little or no data-based justification. But for the more reputable and pediatrician-favored screening tools (the ones that have been designed specifically based on data collected for that purpose), this number is often just another simple percentile: the ninetieth.

Let's go back to that same hypothetical playgroup. More simple statistics dictate that one baby will be in the "red flag" range for an earlier milestone like rolling over, which should start at four months. So in a small playgroup of ten typically developing six-month-olds, *half of them* won't be able to sit without help, and one will be *officially delayed* and not even be able to roll over.

There's also an even more fundamental issue with the data we use to create developmental averages and red-flag ages, and it's a doozy. The majority of studies on milestones have not included anything close to a representative sample of children of different races, ethnicities, sexes, genders, and cultural backgrounds. And this does absolutely matter. Recent data is just beginning to show how much variation there is in infant development depending on all these factors. It means that most of the current guidelines we have, even the ones that are based on a good amount of real-world science, frequently overdiagnose, or even miss, developmental delays for babies in underrepresented groups.

As much as I love to rage against frequently anxiety-provoking guidelines, I'm still a doctor. It's important to remember that developmental cutoffs, no matter how limited they are, no matter how skeptical we need to be when we interpret them, serve a purpose when used correctly. The reality is that they intentionally signal an alarm early, usually much earlier than there's an actual problematic delay, to make sure that we don't miss anything. This is because every developmental problem can be treated much more effectively the earlier it's discovered. And those serious medical conditions that cause delays are even more important to find early and treat. From the perspective of hard science and clinical medicine, it's better to err on the side of caution and be a little conservative. What's the problem with that?

Though there are some parents who seem completely unfazed by milestone madness, able to observe and enjoy developmental achievements without compulsive tracking or undue worry, the increasing trend I see in my personal and professional life is one of mounting anxiety. I'm guilty of per-petuating it myself. Like when I told Arthur's mother at his twelve-month checkup that we should keep a close eye on his language development. Yes, he seemed to understand what people said, could follow simple directions, made good eye contact, and was otherwise growing and developing well. But he hadn't met that critical checklist item of being able to speak at least one word. When I said this, his mom seemed confused. Did I think there was something wrong with him?

I reviewed with her how it was extremely likely that Arthur would start talking in the next few months, and how pedia-tricians just like to catch things as early as possible in case there's an issue that can be treated. But the seeds of anxiety had already been planted. Each of my suggestions seemed only to increase her worry. How about making an appointment to come back in one month? She nodded, but her eyes went wide. I kept going. If he still didn't speak then, I could refer to Early Intervention for an official (and free!) developmental evalua-tion. Her body visibly tensed. In the end, I walked it all back and did my best to reassure her. Arthur would be fine, and we would see him at his fifteen-month visit. I would call to check in and see how everything was going next month, and I was sorry to have added to her worries! We parted on good terms. In six weeks, when I called to follow up, she brightly answered on the first ring. She happily told me that Arthur could now speak *five* words: "mama," "dada," "bottle," "water," and "up." Everything had really been fine all along.

There's a fine line between healthy monitoring and stress-inducing vigilance. So let's divide and conquer: Your pediatrician will do all of the worrying, and you can do all of the enjoying. When I was a brand-new mom, I wish I had been able to realize that my anxious, worst-case-scenario developmental fears were just that: fears. Yes, delays are real, problems are detectable, and developmental screening is important. It's just not your job. You're a loving parent, and you can stay appropriately aware of your baby's growth without letting it interfere with the actual joy of promoting it.

Because it turns out that milestones can be super fun to witness—and nurture—once the stressful noise is removed. Do your best to reframe the entire process and approach your milestone monitoring with curiosity instead of judgment. It will make your social media feeds less stressful, and let you spend playtime enjoying each milestone that is met, not tracking it. The pediatrician well-child visits are scheduled not only to make sure all vaccines are up-to-date (hooray!) but also to let us check up on your baby frequently, over time, and early on. You'll bring all your questions and concerns to those visits, and your pediatrician will be able to decide next steps. And if you have any amount of worry, no matter how small, in the months, weeks, and days before your next well-child visit, just call! Pediatricians love to have extra visits in between routine checkups to give special attention to any and every parental concern, milestone madness included.

THE BOTTOM LINE

5 out of 5 Pediatrician Parents Agree

- Milestones aren't set in stone. Pediatricians use them as rough guidelines to make sure babies are generally on track and that there isn't a major medical problem going on.

- These major problems are almost always seen when multiple milestones are delayed, and usually when they occur in multiple categories (fine motor, gross motor, language, and social/problem-solving).

- Milestones are averages, so for many assessments this means that, by definition, half of babies will be "delayed" on any given milestone. Even "red flag" delays are usually based on the 90th percentile, meaning 1 in 10 babies will have a "concerning" delay.

- It's important for pediatricians to track milestones and start to "worry" earlier than necessary so they don't miss anything. Delays are diagnosed and treated best when found early on.

- However, *you* don't need to worry about this! Focus on playing with your baby and enjoying their development—and leave the tracking and testing to your pediatrician.

19

THAT'LL TEACH YOU

. . . .

Staying Sane in a World Filled with Baby Classes and Extracurriculars

With music classes, baby gyms, and even baby sign language, there are endless ways to spend time and money "educating" your infant. Promoting development is certainly important, but when school seems to start at birth, it's clear that this new obsession with early learning has gone overboard. When, if at all, should you spend time and money on baby activities, and which are worthwhile?

My daughter started day care after we moved from Michigan to New York, and I was nervous to transition from her incredible nanny to an unknown childcare center, even in pre-pandemic times. My hesitation was short-lived, however; within weeks, it became clear that her teachers were incredible, doing what could only be described as a superhuman job of herding eight toddlers through a day's worth of scheduled enrichment activities. My daughter experienced some combination of music classes, gym classes, arts and crafts, story time, sensory play, and outside recess in addition to her meals, snacks, diaper changes, and naps on a daily basis. I shared photos with grandparents, images of my ten-month-old with a soccer ball and a caption explaining how she was working on gross motor development. She and I arrived home equally exhausted from our respective days of work and play, and each morning she woke up eager for more. By the time she turned twelve months, not a weekend went by without her grabbing my hand and taking me to her stroller, signaling before she even had the words that five days of "school" wasn't nearly enough. I had clearly made a great choice.

My daughter's preschool, if you haven't already guessed, was a specific type—the pricey, corporate-branded kind that boasts educational activities, trained teachers, and fancy apps to check in on your baby at all times. I chose mine out of availability and geographical convenience, so while I wanted a reputable center with good credentials, the enrichment activities really were a surprising bonus. The question, then, is: Would I have chosen a center just for this curriculum? Or, if I had chosen a full-time nanny, would a day's worth of baby classes have been worth the money?

A quick review of the basics of development in the first year of life. "Basic" is the key word. These early days are the busiest in your baby's brain, as they constantly create and refine neural connections. The neuroscience is indeed quite complicated, but the achievements—and the environmental stimuli they need to experience in order to reach them—are (adorably) simple. To have a good foundation for language learning, your baby doesn't need to accomplish much in their first year. They'll learn how to process spoken words and gestures, and to communicate through facial expressions, movements, cries, smiles, mimicry, and sounds. Their only task for emotional development is to learn how to explore the world around them, sort through what is and isn't safe, learn who they can trust (you!) and who they prefer to be around (also you!). Their motor development will progress swiftly from not moving purposefully at all to rolling, sitting, scooting, grabbing objects, or maybe even taking their first few steps. So while your baby's brain is absolutely in overdrive, there really isn't much else that they need from outside their own miraculous mind to get them where they need to be.

When I say there's "not much else," I mean it. The only thing your baby *needs* to grow and thrive is a safe and interactive environment. It's something that can be built almost anywhere that there are loving people around them (and a few very bare-bones playthings). There's no specific brand of childcare that's better or best, and any compassionate caretaker (like my daughter's incredible day care teachers or nannies) can create an environment in which your baby can explore their world. The specific activities are unimportant. The only requirements to any infant's daily schedule are socializing with others; having space to crawl, scoot, and roll around; hearing language and sounds (we love you, early literacy!); and having a few objects to pick up, put in their mouth, and bang around.

That's really it. Any reputable childcare center will provide these, and I can confidently say that there is no need for kids in day care to engage in extracurriculars. If you go the nanny/caretaker route—or stay home to care for your baby yourself—there's also no need to stress. Without the built-in socialization and enrichment of day care, the pressure mounts higher to spend even more money on infant education. Yet the evidence shows that replacing a pricey baby gym membership with a local library's worth of story time and free play in the children's section (or an outdoor, pandemic-friendly playgroup) is an excellent choice. Music, gym, yoga, and even baby math classes will provide the exact same developmental opportunities as any unstructured baby get-together with age-appropriate toys and engaged caretakers. It's not that there's anything wrong with these activities! There are plenty of other potential benefits, like giving you opportunities to socialize with other parents, or simply adding a fun activity to the day's schedule. If you want to spend that thirty dollars per hour on a newborn music class, rock on! But you also should know that opting for (literally) free play will not doom your child to a life of educational disadvantage.

The less-is-more, play-is-enough approach to parenting crystallized during the pandemic—for me personally and for countless other parents. The sudden onset of childcare closures, isolation, and a world of covid-precautions made in-person, structured play less accessible than ever. Parents like me learned how incredibly resilient children are, and how they can reach their full potential without the enrichment activities we have become so used to. With day care closed, and socialization initially limited, it was hard not to feel like the entire weight of my daughter's development rested on my shoulders. But I quickly saw how she was able to adapt, and how I was able to follow her lead. I recall one day of #stayathome parenting where we explored the outdoors together. It was remarkable to see her create her own learning experience through play, pointing to animals, plants, finding shapes and colors, and expanding her imagination. Did I know that some leaves are shaped just like stars? It's a particularly fond memory from a particularly dark time, and a reminder of the experiences one can find when structure and expectations loosen.

I also remind myself of the fact that traditional education is merely one way for children to grow and thrive. This is especially true for babies and toddlers. It wasn't until just a few decades ago that formalized curricula for young kids (let alone babies) were the norm. To put it in perspective, just think of all the certifiable geniuses out there who invented vaccines, cured diseases, created art and music, all after a childhood filled only with free play and without a single school class until the first grade!

The first year of life is one of the most overwhelming times. It's also, in many ways, the easiest for promoting development. As a pediatrician and working mother, I assure you that love, attention, and a few playmates are all you need to create a stimulating, enriching environment for your infant. The rest—fancy classes, playgroups, and "educational" activities—are only worth as much as the enjoyment they bring you.

THE BOTTOM LINE

5 out of 5 Pediatrician Parents Agree

- Any infant in day care will have more than enough developmental engagement and stimulation.

- Any loving caretaker who can provide attention is almost all babies need to thrive—an additional activity a few times a week that lets babies socialize with others, especially other kids, is the only other ingredient.

- Your baby is already resilient. If quarantine, childcare closures, or other circumstances arise that temporarily take social visits off the table, they will still grow and thrive.

- Extracurriculars are only as valuable as the enjoyment (or reprieve from being in charge of developmental play) they bring parents.

20

YOUR BABY DOESN'T NEED KOMBUCHA

• •

The Truth about Vitamins, Supplements, and "Alternative" Products

"Immune boosting" supplements, spinal adjustments, essential oils, and assorted herbal remedies. These days, it seems there's a "natural" treatment for every baby woe imaginable. I've seen many parents who assume that over-the-counter, herbal, organic, or any combination of these qualifying labels means that a product is safe. And with so many "alternative" products specifically marketed to infants, I don't blame them. But the reality is that not only are the majority of these remedies ineffective—they also have the potential to cause real harm. Let's review the alphabet of "natural" or so-called alternative baby treatments, from Acupuncture to Zarbee's.

Modern medicine has a huge problem. In an age of increasing dissatisfaction and distrust with our for-profit medical system, many parents express understandable anxiety that there are just too many medications, tests, pokes, and shots these days. It's true. We have more treatments than ever, and people—kids included—visit doctors more frequently. It's a complex issue, and there are times when I agree babies are given medical treatments that they either don't really need (like those acid medicines for reflux) or can even be harmful (like unnecessary antibiotics for probably viral infections). But I'm still a pediatrician, and remain a believer in modern medicine, which has done wonders to help children lead long and healthy lives. There's room for a balanced discussion, understanding that "traditional" medicine has an important role even for the tiniest patients, while acknowledging that overtreating is a real issue.

However, the booming "alternative" market (let's call them Big Nature to match their Big Pharma counterparts) has forced a far less balanced conversation. Why be thoughtful about the risks and benefits of modern medical treatments and make individualized decisions? Instead, Big Nature offers an alternative: Ditch "traditional" medicine altogether and go the route of the "natural." There are now an obscene number of unregulated and risky treatments targeted specifically to anxious parents and their vulnerable babies. You can find them in each chapter of this book: high velocity chiropractic manipulation for breastfeeding, acupuncture for colic, homeopathic teething drops, and plain old "organic" vitamins peddled to parents whose kids already eat nutritious and complete baby-led diets. I meet so many new parents, often coming off a "medicalized" birth and recovery period, who just want to do what's best, most "gentle" for their baby's colic. Why shouldn't they buy the "natural" gas drops located right between the organic diaper creams and fragrance-free wipes at their local pharmacy?

Many pediatricians take a relatively black-and-white approach to this topic. Unregulated products are dangerous, untested, and with no clear benefit. The underlying sentiment is dead-on. I have enough stories to scare me off unregulated treatments for the rest of my life (and my daughter's as well). I'll never forget Abby, a ten-month-old girl with a very serious illness that caused her blood cells to attack her body. The result was a body constantly inflamed, and severe organ damage that required frequent hospitalizations for intensive IV medications. When I saw her, she was in acute liver failure. It took weeks to crack the case—why was her liver failing when all her other organs were doing so much better? Her mother, so loving and so desperate to help her however she could, had taken the advice of a trusted relative and given her daughter turmeric. Turmeric is a plant purported to have magical anti-inflammatory and healing properties. But it can also cause severe liver injury, and it had never crossed Abby's mother's mind that there could be serious side effects. In fact, she was so sure that "herbal" meant "harmless" that it didn't even occur to her to mention this treatment until we probed deeper.

This extreme example was followed by many others. One mother applied so much lavender essential oil to her baby's eczema that the child ended up developing hormonal abnormalities; a teething infant developed belladonna poisoning from unregulated homeopathic teething drops (other babies died, but Hyland refused to recall its product). Another baby was drunk on kombucha, a supplement touted for its intestinal and brain health benefits, but whose active ingredients include caffeine and alcohol.

While I understand, as a pediatrician, wanting to simply say no to any nontraditional remedy, the reality is that taking a hardline stance against anything is never the right choice. I know that you're smart and caring, and you deserve a complete breakdown of what safety information we do and don't have for natural treatments. It is true, however, that the majority of "natural" and "alternative" products are unregulated. It's also true, just as we went over in our vaccine discussion, that natural does not mean safer, and that there's no meaningful difference between "natural" and "chemical" products. You see, the thing about molecules is that it doesn't really matter where they came from. The human body handles the active ingredient from a tea, plant, oil, or tincture in exactly the same way that it handles a synthesized compound designed to mimic the plant it was discovered in (which accounts for the majority of all pharmaceutical treatments). It may be easy to trick our minds, but our bodies see everything that we put into them as medicine. And all medicines have risks and benefits. Approaching alternative products with as much, if not more, skepticism than any other medicine, is definitely the way to go.

Let's start by going over the framework I use when counseling parents on whether or not a nontraditional treatment makes sense. If you use these guiding questions in your discussion with your own pediatrician, and for self-reflection, you'll be able to make the smartest, safest choices for your baby.

Does My Baby Need Treatment at All?

Even before COVID-19 swept the globe, parents found themselves with an endless sea of products marketed as having some sort of "immune boosting" property. They also found—and still find—countless advertisements suggesting that their infants required specific supplements in order to grow and develop. In short, to sell something, a company needs to convince you that something is missing, that your baby has a problem that needs to be fixed.

The reality, however, is that the most important ingredients for your little one to grow, thrive, fight illnesses, and develop a strong immune system are already things you're providing. Breast milk (plus vitamin D drops) and/or formula, a varied diet of solid foods, a full set of vaccines, and a relatively active lifestyle are all the overwhelming majority of babies ever need to reach their full potential and become the pinnacle of infant fitness. Nutritional deficiencies of macro- and micronutrients are exceedingly rare, and your pediatrician will be the first to let you know if there's a concern.

When approaching any alternative remedy, the first step is to ask yourself: Is something wrong? Does my baby need to take medicine? Remember that everything that your baby ingests *is* a medicine and comes with risk, no matter how small. It's not possible to say that something is necessary, effective, or important without also acknowledging that this makes it, by definition, a medical treatment with real risks and benefits. For now, there's no evidence that any available supplement helps infants when given routinely. Same for the countless unregulated gas-drops, colic tinctures, and assorted remedies for everyday baby fuss. While it's easy to take a "why not?" approach to these seemingly low-risk supplements and give them just in case, science (and common sense) don't support this.

Starting the discussion with the first, fundamental question of whether your baby needs treatment has been a complete game changer for me and for so many parents. I remember my visit with Erin, a vibrant nine-month-old in for her routine checkup. We reviewed her medications, and they confirmed she wasn't taking any. Just some gripe water for gas pain. I paused and tried what was then a new approach for me. No lectures on regulation and safety, just questions. Why did they think Erin needed medicine for her gas? They were surprised—in their minds, they weren't giving a medication, just an over-the-counter, natural supplement.

The conversation flowed easily from there, discussing how anything that promised relief was a medicine, that all medications have risks and benefits, but that some medicines were better understood and regulated than others. We learned together that this brand was reluctant to have its products studied and did have some bad effects reported. Did they want me to look up some other options that might be safer to try? No, they decided, the drops worked a little, but honestly, Erin's gas pain wasn't so bad. They had just been using it because it came highly recommended from a friend. We decided we'd check back in a month and see how things were going, if anything needed treatment at that time, and take it from there.

Who Is Telling Me That My Baby Needs This Treatment?

Hear about it from a friend? Did they see it on their social media feed? Maybe it wasn't an actual #ad, but there was a link that gave the promoter a commission—or maybe there's a partnership they didn't even disclose. In the world of the health influencer, it's harder than ever to fully understand the motivation behind any parenting recommendation. Sorting through supplements, treatments, and "holistic" options for your little one has become almost impossible. Is it genuine advice? Less scrupulous, predatory advertising? Something in between? It's challenging for scrollers, no matter how savvy, to know for sure.

Even if the product is something the promoter truly believes in, it's hard to be completely objective when financial gains are at stake. Online, I refuse to promote products for profit (even ones I genuinely adore) because I know that it will cloud my objectivity. It's why in medicine our days are filled with financial disclosure forms, investigations into conflicts of interest, and constant introspection into how we can provide the best, most honest information possible without succumbing to undue influence. So keep your expectations high for the integrity of traditional medicine and health-care corporations, and raise them just as high for anyone promoting a "natural" product.

Has This Treatment Been Tested? How and By Whom?

The simple truth is that any "alternative" remedy won't come with a lot of good science behind it. Some of that is Big Nature at work, but some of it is also traditional medicine's fault. We've been reluctant to study alternative products for a variety of reasons (Big Pharma, racism, xenophobia, arrogance, funding), and it's something we're trying to fix. There are more and more studies to determine if these treatments are safe and effective, and we have better evidence to guide our recommendations each day. The reality, though, is that this data is still sparse, and even when we do have studies, it's much harder to draw conclusions about safety and efficacy because of how much variety we see between different practices and the composition of different substances. In the end, it's still challenging to find high-quality pediatric evidence for the majority of alternative treatments, especially for infants.

For supplements and "natural" remedies, a lack of appropriate regulation also makes safety a real concern. Most of these products have, through very clever lobbying, been able to classify themselves as "dietary supplements" and escape the rigorous FDA review that "pharmaceuticals" must go through. This means that these products go through exactly zero external review of safety beyond their own, conflict-of-interest-filled testing. I can't imagine anyone (myself included!) feeling comfortable with a traditional pharmaceutical company's safety approval process consisting of self-proclaiming their own safety to the FDA. And there is just as much potential for improper regulation leading to real harm when it comes to so-called dietary supplements. Just ask Jack's mom, who had chosen to focus on behavioral therapy for his ADHD treatment rather than taking a prescribed stimulant medication. Things were going well until a few months after starting an attention-boosting, over-the-counter supplement a friend recommended. When his mood started worsening and his kidney function took a slight turn for the worse (Jack had a rare but treatable kidney condition, so we checked his blood work routinely), we were initially puzzled. Until we read the full ingredients label from his fancy new supplement and found that caffeine and lithium, two kidney-damaging, mood-disrupting substances, were the first two ingredients.

The lack of safety and efficacy data is the main reason that so many pediatricians prefer to just say no to untested infant products altogether. If you do decide that an unregulated product is something you want to explore, make sure to be even more cautious, even more skeptical, and even more critical of the safety and efficacy claims you see. With all that in mind, you can start the conversation with your pediatrician also knowing that there are some nontraditional products that are safer and/or more effective than others.

For Your Consideration: Alternative Treatments That Are Reasonable to Consider Giving to Your Infant

1. Essential oils

We're still lacking enough data to say that using essential oils and aromatherapy in infancy has consistent, meaningful benefits. But as long as you keep these items safely stored when not in use (I have in fact seen a toddler in the emergency room with "essential oil overdose" in my pediatric residency!), there's low potential for harm. Aromatherapy is something we offer to pediatric patients in the hospital, and even something that's being embraced by health-care providers in the neonatal intensive care units to help soothe premature infants.

Just keep your aromatherapy as aromatherapy. I discourage topical use for a variety of reasons. Babies have a large amount of skin surface area for their size, and it's easy to absorb anything that gets placed on them (and many of the ingredients in these oils, like lavender, can absolutely change a baby's biology when taken up into the bloodstream). Baby skin is also sensitive, and putting anything on it other than fragrance-free wash and dermatologist-approved ointments can get very irritating very fast. I also advise against using diffusers and other fragrance dispensers. Kids with asthma-like breathing physiology find this very irritating, and as a rule, inhaling any unregulated, aerosolized substance can damage developing lungs.

2. Gas drops

Like Erin's parents, you'll want to ask yourself if there's something going on with your fussy baby that really needs fixing. If so, trying a "gas drop" that you buy from a reputable vendor (such as your local pharmacy, and not off someone's social media feed or from a company that will mail directly to you) is reasonable to try. The same caveats apply. You'll want to chat with your pediatrician to review whatever data is available, make sure the company has a good reputation without serious safety issues or recalls, and look through the ingredients to make sure there are no red flags (like those "cramp-preventing" hormones in many colic treatments, or "homeopathic" doses of actual poisons such as belladonna). Some parents swear by simethicone, gripe water, and other probably safe, possibly effective options. Engage in some introspection, give your pediatrician a call, and reevaluate the risks vs. benefits in real time as your baby grows and responds to your treatment.

3. Probiotics

Probiotics are one of the so-called alternative remedies that are quickly being embraced by the world of traditional medicine. There's enough biological plausibility and compelling data to suggest that a variety of babies with a variety of conditions will benefit from their use. The most notable cases are kids with inflammatory bowel disease, little ones who are taking antibiotics, and emerging data on potential benefits for colicky infants. If you stick to a reputable vendor (or even replace a supplement with a probiotic-containing yogurt as you start your solid food adventures)—and talk to your pediatrician—there's a good chance that giving your infant probiotics is a safe choice.

4. Infant massage

No, your baby doesn't need a full day at the spa or a deep-tissue treatment. But gentle infant massage is a common and almost certainly safe practice. It's what many neonatal intensive care units routinely provide to their patients to promote growth and development. There's no data to suggest this should be a requirement for every infant, premature or not. Practices also vary widely, and I remain highly skeptical of anyone offering pricey lessons or even in-person sessions as some sort of baby health necessity. When there is a musculoskeletal issue that requires therapeutic touch—like torticollis or increased body tone—physical therapy is the only way to go. But if you'd like to give gentle massage a try (with some common sense, making sure to avoid needlessly kneading any imagined newborn knots), it's a fine option to consider.

Hard Pass: Your Baby Truly Does Not Need Kombucha (or Any of These Other Treatments)

1. Acupuncture

There is decent evidence for acupuncture, even in certain pediatric populations—just not for infants. As we reviewed earlier, it doesn't work for colic (and seems to only make it worse). This means that the potential harms, no matter how rare, easily outweigh the not-yet-existent benefits.

2. Unregulated supplements, herbs, teas, tablets, and anything else your baby ingests

I've said it here, and in almost every chapter before this, but it bears repeating: Anything your baby ingests is a medicine. Untested medicines are dangerous, and untested supplements, tablets, herbs, teas, and drops are just as dangerous. It's okay to be super selective about the substances that you let your baby put in their mouth. Your baby doesn't need kombucha, and they also don't need teething necklaces, colic drops, dietary supplements, or anything your social media feed is trying to convince you to buy.

3. Chiropractic adjustments

In Chapter 7 we parsed through the important difference between craniosacral therapy, infant

massage, and high-velocity chiropractic manipulation. The data is limited for the first two, but
the potential for harm is low as long as you keep
common sense front and center. What common
sense—and real life—absolutely advise against?
High-velocity chiropractic manipulation. I've
seen countless families explore this treatment for
all sorts of infant woes including breastfeeding
difficulties, colic, reflux, and even as a routine
preventive therapy. But it's absolutely a hard no
for me. Infant chiropractic adjustments not only
have zero proven benefit, but messing with their
tiny spine can also truly be dangerous.

The allure of the natural can no longer be ignored. As a new
parent, you'll be bombarded with "alternative" products
from the very first moments of your baby's life. It's impossible
to sort through it all without some basic guidance, and I hope
you can use my framework to partner with your pediatrician
and make the safest choices possible. Your baby definitely
does not need kombucha, but it's totally okay to explore certain alternative remedies with their doctor and incorporate
them into the rest of their medical care and health.

THE BOTTOM LINE

5 out of 5 Pediatrician Parents Agree

- Everything that you put in or on your baby's body is a medicine. There is no difference between "natural" and "chemical."

- Since "natural" and "alternative" remedies are medicines, they can have real benefits. Unfortunately, many of these remedies haven't gone through enough scientific testing to know that they are safe to use.

- There are real side effects, even for these "natural" medicines. Sometimes these are serious and life-threatening.

- If you're considering an alternative treatment for your baby, ask yourself if the symptoms are something you'd be comfortable giving a "real medicine" to treat. If not, then it's not worth the risk to your baby. If so, talk to your pediatrician first to make sure there aren't any dangerous side effects.

- Data is limited, but there's enough evidence and science to suggest that aromatherapy, massage, gas drops, and probiotics are reasonable to consider for your infant. High-velocity chiropractic adjustments, unregulated supplements, and acupuncture, on the other hand, should just be avoided.

EPILOGUE

●●●●●●●●●●●●●●●●●●●●●●●●●●●●●●●●●●●●●●

A Send-Off into
Safe and Sane Toddlerhood

Congratulations! Not just on getting to the end of this book, but on being an amazing parent already. You clearly love your baby and are going to do everything you need to do to create a warm, supportive, nurturing environment. There's no need to ditch science, but there's also no need to ignore common sense. I hope you feel fully confident that the first year of your little one's life will be filled with maximal joy, safety, and sanity.

Bask in this accomplishment. Did you bask? Great. Now let's take a sneak peek at what's to come: toddlerhood.

Spoiler alerts abound. No need to rush ahead through the mommy blogs; just do your best to stay present in every moment of your baby's precious first year. Here's all the fun that's to come in the toddler years. Stick with me and you'll be able to tackle it with (relative) ease.

#TimesUp for Time-Out

In an age of "snowplow" parenting (in which parents attempt to push away all of life's obstacles from a child's path, to assure success), we are increasingly unwilling to tolerate our children

303

being even in temporary discomfort. We'll explore how centuries of research in behavioral psychology and resilience training, combined with a loving, empathic approach, can create a framework for dealing with tantrums, biting, and everyday toddler meltdowns.

Toilet Training

No, quarantine and #workfromhome did not mean we miraculously had the energy and motivation to take advantage of our isolation and follow a strict potty-training regimen. And it turned out just fine.

Milk Money

Just as you put away the last bottles, pump parts, and infant-feeding accessories, your social media feed flashes an ad for toddler formula: Organic, plant-based, non-toxic, expensive, and necessary! Nope. We'll debunk the never-ending myths, promotions, and products that needlessly stress toddler parents. It's time to optimize your little one's nutrition without losing any money, time, or sanity.

Your Toddler Still Doesn't Need Kombucha

Same rules apply, but now even more confusing marketing is heading your way. Don't worry, we'll get through it together.

I Screen, You Screen, We All Still Screen

With even more freedom comes even more responsibility. We'll learn how to navigate an increasingly screen-filled world in a way that continues to embrace the reality of screen-ubiquity, and with the dose of moderation and healthy boundaries that your developing toddler's brain needs.

Toddler Sleep Regression

Just months from your hard-earned sleep training win, this terrible sleep rite of passage rears its ugly head. We'll work together to make sure it's as short-lived and painless as possible.

Parenting challenges never go away, but they do change. Parenting is an amazing journey—that first year is just the beginning!—and this pediatrician-mom will be here for all of it.

ACKNOWLEDGMENTS

"**S**o, when's your book coming out?"

What started as a sort of inside joke (as I answered an increasing number of questions from new parent friends, and friends of friends, and friends of friends of friends), led to a yearslong process of making *Parent Like a Pediatrician* a reality. It's surreal. And I simply could not have done any of it without the incredible people who supported me at every step.

Thank you to Stuart Reid for not only being the first to suggest that writing this book was something I should seriously pursue but also for showing me exactly how to make that dream possible. Thank you to Sara Manning Peskin, the inspiring physician mom and author and friend who also edited my attempt at a proposal and helped me find my agents.

To my agents, Justin Brouckaert and Todd Shuster, I'm still amazed that you knew my passion for realistic, safe parenting advice could turn into this powerhouse of a book. Thank you for pushing me at every step of the way and allowing me to find this singular voice as a parenting author. Justin, I can't get over just how many back-and-forth edits you patiently went through with my proposal. I will always be grateful for the time you took to help me shape my writing for the better.

Thank you to everyone at Kensington for believing in this book unconditionally and integrally, often more than I believed in it myself. To Denise Silvestro, my phenomenal editor, who helped this first-time author wade through the exciting (and sometimes overwhelming) process of actually writing a book. To Ann Pryor, who has spent so much effort in publicizing this book and is the reason it will reach the audience that needs it.

This book comes from the deepest parts of my being. It stems from my true sense of self, a feeling of worth and love that I maintain through my family and friends. And I'm so lucky to be loved and supported by so many. I can only "parent like a pediatrician" because of the parenting I have myself been fortunate enough to receive. To my parents, who showed me from the very beginning that unconditional love for a child is simply an expectation. To my mom, a badass doctor-mom herself who made raising four children look easy. There has never been a more devoted mother and I continue to use your parenting as a source of inspiration. To my dad, who actively loved and supported his children before society routinely expected this of fathers.

Thank you to each and every member of my large, warm, messy, and wonderful family who continue to support me in all that I do. To my three incredible brothers, who outshine me so spectacularly that I am filled with far more pride than jealousy. To my aunts, uncles, cousins, grandparents, nieces, nephews. Growing up alongside so many of you is what helped me become the person I am today. Thank you for always being there for me, and for bringing new and wonderful people into our family. To Nana and Poppop, I hope it's always been clear how much of who I am has been shaped by you, and how grateful I am. Nana, your legacy shines through the endless accomplishments of the family you created. You were the mother of mothers, our matriarch, and my biggest cheerleader. I miss you every day, and I know you would have loved this book.

To my amazing friends, who continue to inspire and encourage me daily. Hilary Haimes, Katelyn O'Connor, Susanna O'Kula—med school may be over, but you'll always be my "girls" crew. Avital Fischer, my forever work spouse. Katharine Magliocco, I would be lost without you. Thank you for being my number one fan, unpaid brand manager, life coach, and true friend. Emily Rassel, my one-time co-parent and all-time pediatrician-mom idol. Phoebe Danziger, my mind-twin who started me on this writing journey way back when and who continues to inspire and intimidate me in the best of ways.

Thank you to the experts who so graciously shared their brilliance with me and helped me provide evidence-based guidance in this book. Melissa Glassman, Ellie Erickson, Cristina Fernandez, and countless other physician colleagues and role models who showed me how pediatrician parents can speak up and make a difference.

Like so many parents, I wouldn't be able to do anything without the incredible efforts of childcare workers. Priscila, thank you for helping me raise my daughter to be the wonderful person she is. I couldn't have accomplished any of this without knowing that she was loved and safe in your care. Michelle, the original nanny, thank you for giving us our foundation.

I share my own mental and physical health struggles throughout this book so others will feel empowered to get the help they need. Thank you to my own health-care team. To

Dr. Katie Pasque, without whom I literally wouldn't be alive, I still look to you as a model for my work both as a physician and also as a supporter of parents. To my own psychiatrist and therapist, thank you for getting me through everything.

And above all, this book is dedicated to the loves of my life. To my husband, thank you for being you. You are the best partner I could ever have hoped for, and a greater father than I ever could have imagined existed. And to my daughter, whom I love more than words can ever express. Everything I do is to make the world a better place for you. You are my light, my joy, my proudest accomplishment. The greatest privilege and pleasure in my life is being your mommy.

INDEX

Pepcid, 143

Period of PURPLE Crying,
138–40

peripartum depression, 127

pertussis, 60

petroleum jelly, 80, 81, 82, 84,
87–88

Pfizer COVID-19 vaccine,
165–66

phenylketonuria (PKU), 12,
31–32

physical examination, 11–12,
26–29

picky eaters, 255, 260–61, 263

play gyms, 48, 281

play mats, 48

pneumonia, 61, 156

polio, 159, 163–64

polysaccharide, 162

polysorbate 80, 169

poop, 70–77
    author's experience, 70,
    71–72
    colors of, 70–73
    constipation, 71, 73–75
    diarrhea, 75–76, 77
    Newborn Checklist, 12,
    29–30
    schedule, 73–76, 77

preservatives, 169–71

Prilosec, 143

probiotics, 148, 297–98

products, 37–53. *see also specific
products*
    author's experience, 38–39
    cost considerations, 40–43
    items not needed, 47–49
    items to purchase before
    baby arrives, 43–45
    items to purchase later,
    45–47
    safe sleep, 39, 43–44, 49–
    50, 95, 98–99, 103–4
    safety considerations,
    42–43, 49–52, 53
    safety recalls, 38–39
    warning labels, 52, 53

purees and cereals, 255–60, 268

quick flashlight test, 30–31

racial disparities, 129–30, 277

Raising Readers, 200

rash. *see* diaper rash

Reach Out and Read, 199–200

reading, 198–204
    best books, 202–3, 204
    bilingualism and, 223–24
    importance of, 199–201

recombinant, 162

red stool, 71

reflux, 136, 143–47, 152
    remedies, 144–46
    sleep and, 102, 145